Caregiving in the Illness Context

Other Palgrave Pivot titles

Alastair Ager and Joey Ager: Faith, Secularism, and Humanitarian Engagement: Finding the Place of Religion in the Support of Displaced Communities

Øyvind Kvalnes: Moral Reasoning at Work

Neema Parvini: Shakespeare and Cognition: Thinking Fast and Slow through Character

Rimi Khan: Art in Community: The Provisional Citizen

Amr Yossef and Joseph Cerami: The Arab Spring and the Geopolitics of the Middle East: Emerging Security Threats and Revolutionary Change

Sandra L. Enos: Service-Learning and Social Entrepreneurship in Higher Education: A Pedagogy of Social Change

Fiona M. Hollands and Devayani Tirthali: MOOCs in Higher Education: Institutional Goals and Paths Forward

Geeta Nair: Gendered Impact of Globalization of Higher Education: Promoting Human Development in India

Geoffrey Till (editor): The Changing Maritime Scene in Asia: Rising Tensions and Future Strategic Stability

Simon Massey and Rino Coluccello (editors): Eurafrican Migration: Legal, Economic and Social Responses to Irregular Migration

Duncan McDuie-Ra: Debating Race in Contemporary India

Andrea Greenbaum: The Tropes of War: Visual Hyperbole and Spectacular Culture

Kristoffer Kropp: A Historical Account of Danish Sociology: A Troubled Sociology

Monika E. Reuter: Creativity – A Sociological Approach

M. Saiful Islam: Pursuing Alternative Development: Indigenous People, Ethnic Organization and Agency

Justin DePlato: American Presidential Power and the War on Terror: Does the Constitution Matter?

Christopher Perkins: The United Red Army on Screen: Cinema, Aesthetics and The Politics of Memory

Susanne Lundin: Organs for Sale: An Ethnographic Examination of the International Organ Trade

Margot Finn and Kate Smith (editors): New Paths to Public Histories

Gordon Ade-Ojo and Vicky Duckworth: Adult Literacy Policy and Practice: From Intrinsic Values to Instrumentalism

DOI: 10.1057/9781137558985.0001

palgrave▶pivot

Caregiving in the Illness Context

Tracey A. Revenson
Professor of Psychology, Hunter College and the Graduate Center, City University New York, USA

Konstadina Griva
Associate Professor of Health Psychology, National University of Singapore, Singapore

Aleksandra Luszczynska
Professor of Psychology, University of Social Sciences and Humanities, Poland

Val Morrison
Professor of Health Psychology, Bangor University, UK

Efharis Panagopoulou
Assistant Professor of Health Psychology, Aristotle University, Greece

Noa Vilchinsky
Lecturer in Rehabilitation Psychology, Bar Ilan University, Israel

Mariët Hagedoorn
Professor of Health Psychology, University of Groningen, the Netherlands

palgrave macmillan

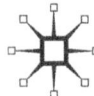

Copyright © Tracey A. Revenson, Konstadina Griva, Aleksandra Luszczynska, Val Morrison, Efharis Panagopoulou, Noa Vilchinsky and Mariët Hagedoorn 2016

All rights reserved. No reproduction, copy or transmission of this publication may be made without written permission.

No portion of this publication may be reproduced, copied or transmitted save with written permission or in accordance with the provisions of the Copyright, Designs and Patents Act 1988, or under the terms of any licence permitting limited copying issued by the Copyright Licensing Agency, Saffron House, 6–10 Kirby Street, London EC1N 8TS.

Any person who does any unauthorized act in relation to this publication may be liable to criminal prosecution and civil claims for damages.

The authors have asserted their rights to be identified as the authors of this work in accordance with the Copyright, Designs and Patents Act 1988.

First published 2016 by
PALGRAVE MACMILLAN

Palgrave Macmillan in the UK is an imprint of Macmillan Publishers Limited, registered in England, company number 785998, of Houndmills, Basingstoke, Hampshire RG21 6XS.

Palgrave Macmillan in the US is a division of St Martin's Press LLC, 175 Fifth Avenue, New York, NY 10010.

Palgrave Macmillan is the global academic imprint of the above companies and has companies and representatives throughout the world.

Palgrave® and Macmillan® are registered trademarks in the United States, the United Kingdom, Europe and other countries.

ISBN: 978-1-137-55899-2 EPUB
ISBN: 978-1-137-55898-5 PDF
ISBN: 978-1-137-55897-8 Hardback

A catalogue record for this book is available from the British Library.

A catalog record for this book is available from the Library of Congress.

www.palgrave.com/pivot

DOI: 10.1057/9781137558985

Contents

Preface		vi
About the Authors		viii
1	What Is Caregiving and How Should We Study It?	1
2	Caregiving Outcomes	15
3	Caregiving as a Dyadic Process	25
4	The Emotional Experience of Caregiving	38
5	Gender and Caregiving: The Costs of Caregiving for Women	48
6	The Influence of Culture on Caregiving Cognitions and Motivations	64
7	Personality and Caregiving	79
8	Interventions to Support Caregivers	90
References		105
Index		151

Preface

At a recent conference on caregiving that one of us (Noa Vilchinsky) attended, a psychologist told the audience about the first time she led a support group for partners of cancer patients. As is often done, the psychologist started by asking each of them to say something about themselves. Each of the participants gave her or his name and the ill spouse's diagnosis and treatment status. She asked again – same response. It took three more rounds before the caregivers were able to say something about themselves that was not related to their partner's illness.

As the above anecdote illustrates, caregiving can be all consuming. In the past, caregiving for an ill person was short-term, as most people did not survive for long or live to old age. Today, caring for an ill family member is better labeled as a long lasting situation. Perhaps as a result of medical advances people are living longer, albeit often with chronic conditions or disabilities, and families remain the "first responders". Those who take on this unpaid role risk incremental stress, physical strain, competing demands, and financial burdens; at the same time, positive benefits can accrue. Governmental policies may make long-term care or institutionalization prohibitive for many and even if aid were available, many people would not want to institutionalize a family member.

Thus, at some point in our lives, most of us will be asked or needed to assume the caregiver role. We should note, however, that many individuals who provide assistance and support to a loved one with chronic illness or disability do not identify themselves as caregivers, but rather describe what they do in terms of their relationship with the other person: as a partner, child, or close friend.

What factors are related to optimal caregiver adjustment? What types of interventions are most effective and cost-effective at reducing caregiver stress and burden? Despite the ubiquity of this phenomenon, we know relatively little about it. There have been multiple reviews and meta-analyses (e.g., Adelman, Tmanova, Delgado, Dion, & Lachs, 2014; Pinquart, & Sörensen, 2005, 2007, 2011) and hundreds of articles, but they tend to focus on caregivers of elderly adults who are frail or have dementia. A key theme to emerge from systematic reviews is that family care may influence the caregivers' own financial situation, physical and emotional health, and ability to continue to care for the recipient at home. The impact is particularly severe for caregivers of individuals who have complex chronic health conditions (Feinberg et al., 2011).

In this volume we synthesize the research evidence on informal (family) caregiving for those with a serious or chronic physical illness or health challenge. Much of this work has been conducted with cancer populations so that emphasis will be evident in many chapters. We also bring in the idea that there are positive outcomes to be gained from caregiving that may offset some of the stressful aspects. After presenting an integrated theoretical framework for caregiving research, we discuss how caregiving affects physical health and emotional well-being and how it should be studied as a dyadic phenomenon between caregiver and care recipient. We then look at several determinants and moderators of caregiver outcomes – emotions, gender, culture, and personality. The volume concludes with a chapter on evidence-based interventions and a challenge for future research.

This volume is the culmination of a meeting of the authors in January 2015 in Thessaloniki, Greece, funded by a network grant from the European Health Psychology Society (EHPS) to Noa Vilchinsky, Tracey A. Revenson, and Val Morrison. The initial idea for a network originated at the Annual Meeting of EHPS in 2013 in Bordeaux, France. For these opportunities and for launching of this network, we are indebted to EHPS. We applaud Rebecca Cipollina for her indispensable help with searching literature, editing, references, and fact-checking, and to the Pleiades – for their luminosity and inspiration.

About the Authors

Konstadina Griva is Associate Professor of Health Psychology at National University of Singapore (NUS). She is a chartered psychologist and a health services researcher whose research is on chronic disease management and measurement. She teaches on the undergraduate/graduate psychology program of NUS and provides training for healthcare professionals.

Mariët Hagedoorn is Professor of Health Psychology in the Department of Health Psychology at the University Medical Center, University of Groningen (UMCG), the Netherlands. Her research focuses on couples coping with illness. She teaches Health Psychology in the Research Master Psychosocial and Clinical Epidemiology, the Graduate School, and the BSc at the UMCG.

Aleksandra Luszczynska is Professor of Psychology at the University of Social Sciences & Humanities, Poland, and associate research professor at the Trauma, Health, & Hazards Center, University of Colorado, USA. She is past president of Health Psychology Division, International Association of Applied Psychology and the editor-in-chief of *Anxiety, Stress, & Coping*.

Val Morrison is a Chartered Psychologist and Professor of Health Psychology at Bangor University, Wales, UK, where she is also College Lead for Research with Impact. She is the co-author of a leading European textbook, *An Introduction to Health Psychology*, and teaches the BSc/MSc Psychology courses in the Clinical Health Psychology track.

Efharis Panagopoulou was trained as a health psychologist at Leiden University, the Netherlands. She received a European Leadership Grant to return to Greece to study stress and emotions in healthcare. She is currently the Director of the Personal and Professional Development Program of the Medical School of Thessaloniki, Greece.

Tracey A. Revenson is Professor of Psychology at Hunter College and the Graduate Center, City University of New York. She has authored ten volumes, including the *Handbook of Health Psychology* and *Couples Coping with Stress*. She is a senior associate editor of *Annals of Behavioral Medicine* and *Medicine* and a past president of the Division of Health Psychology of the American Psychological Association. Revenson received the Nathan Perry Award for Career Contributions to Health Psychology in 2013.

Noa Vilchinsky is Lecturer in Rehabilitation Psychology and the Director of the Psycho-cardiology Research Lab, Department of Psychology, Bar Ilan University, Ramat-Gan, Israel. Vilchinsky is also a certified rehabilitation psychologist, and teaches in the Rehabilitation Psychology track for graduate students in the Psychology Department of Bar-Ilan University.

palgrave▸pivot

www.palgrave.com/pivot

1
What Is Caregiving and How Should We Study It?

Revenson, Tracey A., Konstadina Griva, Aleksandra Luszczynska, Val Morrison, Efharis Panagopoulou, Noa Vilchinsky, and Mariët Hagedoorn. *Caregiving in the Illness Context*. Basingstoke: Palgrave Macmillan, 2016. DOI: 10.1057/9781137558985.0004.

Informal (family) caregivers are the backbone of health and social care delivery in countries throughout the world, including developed countries. Providing informal care to ill family members or friends is a growing phenomenon as the population ages, the prevalence of chronic illness increases, and hospitalizations are shorter (National Alliance for Caregiving & AARP, 2015). The anticipated increase in number of caregivers and in the intensity of caregiving already have made caregiving a public health issue (Schulz & Patterson, 2004).

We begin this book with a few statistics: According to a 2012 survey of the Pew Research Center, 30% of the US population performs the role of family caregiver at some point in their lives (Fox & Brenner, 2012). The estimated prevalence of caring for an adult during the past year was 16.6%, or 39.8 million Americans (National Alliance for Caregiving & AARP, 2015). Although it is difficult to come up with a comparable statistic for Europe, in many European countries a slightly greater number report that they are caring for someone aged 65 and older (e.g., 19% in the Netherlands and 21% in Switzerland; Mestheneos, Triantafillou, and the EUROFAMCARE group, 2005). These numbers are only likely to increase in the next quarter century.

Caregiving takes its toll on the caregiver's health. Almost equivocally, caregivers exhibit greater levels of self-reported stress and psychological distress than population norms (Li & Loke, 2013a) and often more than the recipients of care (e.g., Harden et al., 2013a). In a national survey of adult caregivers in the United States, nearly twice as many caregivers (17%) reported their health as fair or poor compared to the national average of 9% (National Alliance for Caregiving & AARP, 2015). Moreover, 35% of those doing the most intense caregiving reported fair or poor health and one-third said that caregiving had made their health worse (Evercare & National Alliance for Caregiving, 2006); 22% of caregivers felt that their health deteriorated as a result of caregiving (National Alliance for Caregiving & AARP, 2015).

Who is providing informal care?

A 2015 US survey (National Alliance for Caregiving & AARP, 2015) estimated that almost six in ten caregivers (56%) are currently caring for a loved one over age eighteen, while more than four in ten (44%) provided care in the past year but are no longer doing so. The vast majority of caregivers are caring for a relative (85%), while the remaining 15% care for a friend, neighbor, or other nonrelative. Nearly half (49%) are providing care for a parent or parent-in-law and another 12% are caring for a spouse. As the caregiver age rises, the likelihood of caring for a spouse also increases. *Who* provides the care differs greatly among European countries, partially based on government policies, on who is reporting caregiving, and how caregiving is defined. In European countries, between 55% and 80% of care for people aged 65 and older was provided by family members (Mestheneos, Triantafillou, and the EUROFAMCARE group, 2005). In Spain 12% of family caregivers were spouse caregivers, in the Netherlands 14%, in the UK 16%, in Poland and the Czech Republic, 21%, while in Finland 43% were spouse caregivers.

Time spent on caregiving

The amount of time providing care is related to burden and distress. It is part of what is considered "objective burden" and interrupts or replaces work, social, and family responsibilities. Informal caregivers spend an average of 24.4 hours per week providing care (National Alliance for Caregiving & AARP, 2015). Depending on the source, between 13% and 23% of family caregivers provide 40 hours of care a week or more (Evercare & National Alliance for Caregiving, 2006). Higher-hour caregivers (over 20 hours per week) are more likely to be female (62%; National Alliance for Caregiving & AARP, 2015) and to report loss of sleep and appetite, increased pain, and headaches. Caregiving is particularly time-intensive for those caring for a spouse or partner (an average of 45 hours a week). The average duration of caregiving is four years, but this, too, varies widely; 24% of caregivers have been providing care for five years or more and 12% have been providing care for ten years or more (National Alliance for Caregiving &AARP, 2015). A study of cancer caregivers found that the average time spent taking care of cancer patients was 8. 8 hours a day (van Ryn et al., 2011), or nearly one-third of every day.

Over 60% of caregivers perceive themselves to be the primary unpaid caregiver, meaning either that they are sole caregivers (47%) or that there are other unpaid caregivers, but they feel that they provide the majority of unpaid care (16%). The 37% of caregivers who labeled themselves are non-primary caregivers includes 12% who share caregiving equally with someone else and 25% who say another caregiver provides most of the unpaid care (National Alliance for Caregiving & AARP, 2015).

DOI: 10.1057/9781137558985.0004

For a substantial proportion of family caregivers, caregiving isn't their only "occupation": Many are employed outside the home. A survey of over 17,000 employees at all levels of a large corporate employer found that 12% reported they provided care to an elder family member or friend (National Alliance for Caregiving, University of Pittsburgh Institute on Aging, & the MetLife Mature Market Institute, 2010). A Gallup poll (2011) of caregivers who worked at least 15 hours a week found that 72% provide care to a parent, often an elderly parent, and about 15% of them care for parents with dementia and the rest a variety of other chronic illnesses. Caregiving is clearly a long-term commitment: Over half have been providing care for three years or more and another 31% for at least a year.

The illness of a family member thrusts other family members, close friends, and sometimes neighbors and work colleagues into a new life situation where the need to provide care redefines daily life and perceptions of the future. The decision to take care of an ill person is not always a choice; in one US surveys, half of informal caregivers reported they felt they had no choice in taking on their caregiving responsibilities (National Alliance for Caregiving & AARP, 2015).

Many (but not all) caregivers experience serious psychological distress. The level of distress is dependent on a combination of multiple factors, including the illness trajectory, treatment phase, characteristics of the caregiving situation and characteristics of the person.

As will be described in detail in the next chapter, caregiving affects mental, physical, and social health in many ways (see also Schulz & Martire, 2004). Although earlier evidence suggested it may be associated with a higher risk of mortality (Schultz & Beach, 1999), more recent epidemiologic studies suggests that providing care to a family member with a chronic illness or disability is not associated with increased risk of death in most cases, and may instead be associated with a modest survival benefit (Brown et al., 2009; Roth, Fredman, & Haley, 2015). Again, the context of the caregiving situation will shape how caregiving affects health and mortality.

The levels of psychological distress reported are not trivial. Nearly all of the caregivers (91%) in a national survey reported that they suffered from symptoms of depression, and that caregiving made their depression worse (Evercare & National Alliance for Caregiving, 2006). In a US national survey, 50% of caregivers considered their situation as posing moderate to high stress. Studies of cancer caregivers have found that between 20% and 50% report clinical levels of depressive symptoms soon after diagnosis and during initial treatment (Kim, Shaffer, Carver, & Cannady, 2014; Kim, Carver, Shaffer, Gansler, & Cannady, 2015).

Defining caregiving

Informal or family caregiving is defined as the behavioral expression of one's commitment to the welfare of another family member (Pearlin, Mullan, Semple, & Skaff, 1990). It usually refers to the provision of unpaid care to another individual in the family, household, or social network that has physical, psychological, or developmental needs. Informal caregivers are often laypersons who take up their roles without formal preparation, adequate knowledge, resources, and skills needed to perform their tasks (Blum & Sherman, 2010; Northouse, Williams, Given, & McCorkle, 2012). This book refers specifically to caregiving that involves care provision in response to a loved one's health challenges or health declines, above and beyond that what is typical within the particular relationship.

The many types of responsibilities placed on caregivers of the chronically ill can make caregiving a complex experience. Sherman, McGuire, Free, and Cheon (2014) list many of the stressors of caregiving. Although their sample was composed of family caregivers for patients with advanced pancreatic cancer, the issues faced apply to any cancer and, in fact, to almost any serious illness (see also National Alliance for Caregiving & AARP, 2015 for frequencies with which caregiver tasks are reported).

First, family caregivers are often called upon to assist with complex medical and nursing tasks. Informal caregivers are often relied upon to monitor adherence to treatment, with some caregivers expected to learn how to deal with complicated treatments (e.g., home-based dialysis), administer medications, provide symptom management (Fletcher, Miaskowski, Given, & Schumacher, 2012), and accompany the ill person to medical visits (Wolff & Roter, 2011). They often negotiate financial and administrative responsibilities, and navigate the intricacies of the healthcare system (Williams, Tisch, Dixon, & McCorkle, 2013). In many countries, formal care resources, for example visiting nurses or physical therapists, are often limited and sporadic; as a result, many caregivers' needs remain unmet (Blum & Sherman, 2010). Second, caregivers provide practical care. Caregiving may include assistance with basic activities of daily living (e.g., buying groceries), personal care (e.g., help with bathing), and helping with administrative tasks or searching medical information. Third, caregivers provide emotional care, including listening to worries and providing companionship. Fulfilling these tasks requires many hours of care and often brings substantial personal, financial, and mental health costs to the caregivers (Schulz & Martire, 2004).

Caregiving as a dynamic process

One can think of caregiving as a journey, punctuated by stages and transitional events. It begins with anticipation for and acquisition of the caregiver role, moving to the everyday performance of tasks and responsibilities, health crises, and eventual exit from the role (Blum & Sherman, 2010). Caregivers may also transition into and out of the role and, over time, the amount and types of assistance they provide will fluctuate. The notion of informal caregiving as a "career" (New York State Office for the Aging, 2012) connotes the way that it can take over a caregiver's life. At the same time, caregiving evolves in both predictable and unintended ways as health challenges unfold and resources change (Aneshensel, Pearlin, Mullan, Zarit, & Whitlatch, 1995). Much of the research, however, takes a "snapshot in time", providing information on caregiving in the present moment.

Distinguishing caregiving from social support

We want to clarify the difference between caregiving and providing social support although the two overlap. The exchange of social support is part of daily life in most intimate relationships. That is, people tend to support significant others at times of stress (e.g., after failing an exam, a conflict with a co-worker). Many tasks that caregivers fulfill could be labeled as providing social support. A caregiver may listen to the worries of the care recipient (i.e., emotional support) or may do household chores (i.e., instrumental support) or provide companionship.

The key differences are that (1) the care provided is above and beyond that what is typical within the particular relationship, (2) a caregiver is usually providing such support over a more extended period of time at a more regular basis, (3) the provision of support or care is usually more unidirectional than bidirectional, and (4) the provision of support is often born out of necessity or a strong feeling of responsibility or obligation, although most caregivers would say they provide care out of love. Being a caregiver may even become one's social identity, while few people would call themselves a support provider. Still it may be difficult to establish whether acts of care should be seen as part of the "normal" exchange of support, or whether it is above and beyond that what is typical within the particular relationship.

In sum, there is something unique about caregiving that differentiates it from the provision of practical or emotional support. In this book, caregiving involves a sense of perceived responsibility that cannot be turned on or off; you get up with the responsibility and you go to bed with it, which may change your identity.

Measurement of caregiving

Studies use very different definitions and measures of caregiving; some do not define the concept at all. In some studies on caregiver outcomes, patients were asked to indicate the person who was most likely to provide care for them when it was needed (e.g., Kim, van Ryn et al., 2015). This may mean that no actual care was provided. In a study of depression among cancer caregivers, the caregivers were nominated by the survivor as "adult family or family-like individual who provided consistent help during the survivors' cancer experience" (Kim et al., 2014, p. 2). Does "consistent" mean the same thing to different people and is it predicated on the relationships (spouse, sister) or whether the caregiver lives in the same residence? Other studies defined the caregiver as the single person most involved in providing assistance and daily care to the patient (e.g., Lee et al., 2015; Nagpal, Heid, Zarit, & Whitlatch, 2015), but it is likely that for seriously ill persons, there is a network of both formal and informal caregivers. It is also possible that the named caregiver may provide only low levels of care or intermittent care. Some studies require that a person provides a minimum amount of care in terms of number of care tasks or hours of care in order to be considered to be a caregiver; other studies measure the amount of care from either caregiver or patient reports (e.g., Lyons, Zarit, Sayer, & Whitlatch, 2002).

The lack of a singular definition of caregiving and of varied measurements of caregiver burden across the literature has consequences for the generalization of findings and comparison between studies (Romito,

Goldzweig, Cormio, Hagedoorn, & Andersen, 2013; Zarit & Reamy, 2013). In this book, we will try, whenever possible, to describe the caregiving context in terms of type and phase of disease, and the way that caregiving has been measured. Chapter 2 presents a table of some selected measures of caregiving.

Theoretical models of caregiving

Many studies of caregiving base themselves on stress process models to pose research questions, measure constructs, and describe the complex interactions between patient characteristics, medical and treatment characteristics, caregiver characteristics, features of the caregiving situation, cognitive stress appraisals of that situation, and intra- and interpersonal resources that determine caregiving outcomes. Although the models differ in important ways, there is a common core that not only examines the direct effects of these predictors to outcomes but also examines both mediation and moderation processes. Most importantly, within these models and for this book, caregiving processes are embedded within the broader sociocultural and temporal contexts (Revenson, 1990, 2003). This will become more evident in later chapters, for example the chapters on gender (Chapter 5), culture (Chapter 6) and personality (Chapter 7). We describe several of the more frequently used models of caregiving and then provide an integrative framework that scaffolds this book.

Transactional stress and coping model

Much of the research on caregiving is based on the stress and coping model (Lazarus & Folkman, 1984). The model was originally developed as a sequel to Lazarus' previous work on psychological (cognitive) appraisals of stress, and expands those ideas to understand how individual coping efforts are shaped by psychological appraisal of stress which, in turn, shape stress-related outcomes. What is key for caregiving is the notion of psychological or perceived stress: The effects of caregiving on the caregiver's health may be less a result of the actual tasks or amount of care and more a result of the appraisals of these tasks and the entire caregiving situation, including the meaning of caregiving for the caregiver's life. This provides the foundation for understanding why different people exposed to "the same" stressor are affected by it in very different ways.

Caregiver stress process model

The caregiver stress process model (Pearlin et al., 1990) is derived from Pearlin's (1989) description of the stress process. It makes a distinction between primary stressors that stem directly from the needs of the patient (e.g., bathing) and secondary stressors (strains) that arise from the caregiving role (e.g., role overload). These primary and secondary stressors are associated with caregiver psychological distress and physical health declines through a number of mediating and moderating psychosocial factors, such as coping resources, economic status, and characteristics of the caregiving context. An important aspect of this model is that multiple factors and mediating processes can lead to caregiver burden and depression.

Both the transactional stress and coping model and the caregiver stress process model focus on individual coping efforts and how they affect caregiver burden and psychological adjustment. In both models, the objective features of the caregiving situation are conceptualized as the stressors.

Caregiver stress and appraisal model

This model (Yates, Tennstedt, & Chang, 1999) addresses what are seen as limitations in the caregiver stress model and incorporates Lazarus and Folkman's (1984) cognitive appraisal with Pearlin et al.'s (1990) model. Most importantly, caregiving burden is considered to be an appraisal not an "objective" stressor (such as hours or types of care required). This distinguishes between objective stressors and subjective burden, the latter being the caregiver's appraisal of the objective situation, i.e., how stressful it is.

Objective burden leads indirectly to negative caregiver outcomes through subjective appraisals of those primary stressors, which, in turn, shape the caregiver's emotional and physical well-being. As such, the caregiver stress and appraisal model addresses the relationship between caregiver and care recipient, a hole in the caregiver stress model.

Developmental–contextual model of dyadic coping

Although not developed specifically with caregiving in mind, Berg and Upchurch's developmental–context model of dyadic coping (2007) brings the three models discussed above together. The model proposes that members of couples confronted with illness (cf. caregivers and care-recipients) mutually influence each other. Appraisals of the illness situation and coping behavior of one person affect not only his or her own adjustment, but also the other person's adjustment. This process of mutual influence may change over time and is affected by the phase of the disease, the life phase of the couple, and the sociocultural (e.g., culture and gender) and proximal (e.g., marital quality and illness condition) context.

An integrative framework for studying caregiving in the illness context

This volume focuses on a particular caregiving context: when the care recipient has a chronic illness or faces a health crisis. Integrating the theoretical models on caregiving, we propose a general framework that can be used to examine the caregiving process in a flexible manner. The framework is presented in Figure 1. A caveat: The framework is neither a theory nor a singular testable model; it is a general structure that can inform more specific theories, research, and clinical practice.

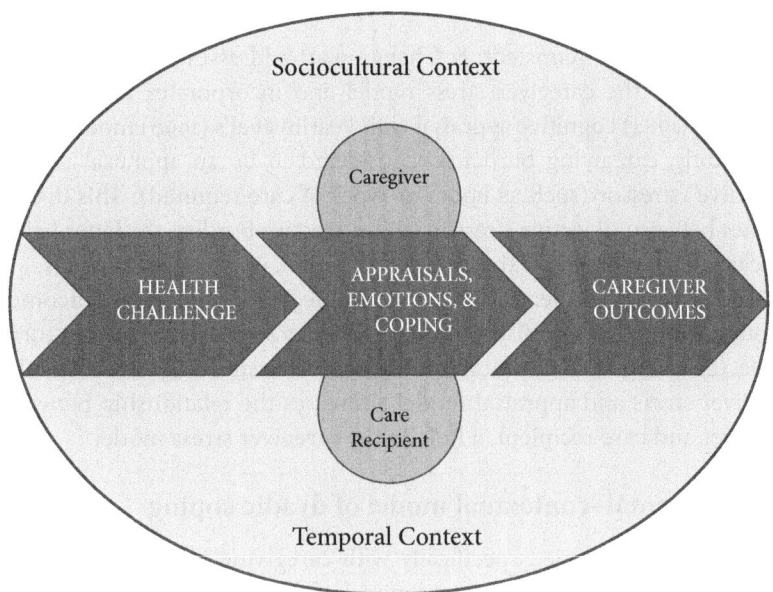

FIGURE 1   *Framework for the caregiving process*

Within the framework, the caregiving situation may be considered as a stressor that poses demands (e.g., objective caregiving tasks and hours of care) as a consequence of the health challenge. The caregiver appraises this situation, perceiving it as stressful or challenging (depending on coping resources), and in turn these perceptions will lead to negative or positive outcomes (e.g., depression or perceived benefits, poorer health; Pinquart & Sorensen, 2007; Harden et al., 2013b; Kim, van Ryn et al., 2015). Although caregiving is enacted in response to a health challenge, it also is moderated by features of that health challenge, such as type of disease, severity, or illness timeline, the caregiver's life phase (age and peer context), caregiver characteristics (e.g., gender, personality dispositions such as attachment orientation and optimism), and the broader sociocultural context (e.g., cultural values about familial responsibility).

In this framework, we conceptualize caregiving as a dyadic interpersonal interaction that involves both the caregiver and the care recipient's perspectives. Moreover, caregiving is not based simply on "objective" or time demands of the situation ("I spent one hour reading to my partner and the whole afternoon driving him to a medical appointment"), but also on the "subjective" perceptions of both members of the dyad ("I now have to do housecleaning tonight when I am exhausted because I spent the day caring for my partner"). The framework incorporates four essential dimensions of caregiving: the health challenge, the temporal context, a dyadic perspective, and a biopsychosocial approach.

Health challenge

Caregiving for an ill person – whether someone with a chronic illness or who is facing a health challenge or health decline – poses unique challenges. For example, the care recipient may need to adhere to a difficult treatment or change health behavior to reduce the risk of intensifying symptoms or to slow down disease progression (prevention context). Alternately the care recipient may be under treatment for a severe, chronic, and possible terminal disease, or may need to deal with the consequences of a chronic disease (rehabilitation context). Each of these health challenges requires some degree of caregiving; that is, the care recipient is assumed to need some degree of help or caregiving.

Illness is broadly defined in the studies we review. Because of its origins in the gerontology literature, the lion's share of research on caregiving focused on studies of caregiving for elderly people or elderly people with dementia. In this volume, we focus more on studies of physical illness in order to cover a broader range of caregiver issues.

The temporal context

The temporal context (Revenson, 1990, 2003) involves both the illness trajectory and the caregiver's life stage. The onset of a disease may be "off-time" in the life cycle. For example, being diagnosed with Parkinson's disease at age 40 is likely to be more difficult than when the disease occurs in later life, which is considered more "on-time" (Neugarten, 1979). With off-time illnesses, neither the patient nor family members are prepared for the changes that illness has on the body or one's daily life.

The trajectory of the illness is also influential. The stage and severity of the illness affect caregiving appraisals, coping, and burden, as does the speed of progression of the illness. For example, in Leventhal's model of illness representations (Leventhal et al., 2012; Chapter 6), whether the illness is seen as acute, chronic, recurrent, or progressive will affect adaptation, and we extend that to caregiving. Moreover, caregiving might be time-limited (post-surgery) or it might be for the rest of the recipient's life, as in the case of a progressive debilitating chronic illness.

A dyadic perspective

Our framework implicitly looks at caregiving as a dyadic relationship (Hagedoorn, Sanderman, Bolks, Tuinstra, & Coyne, 2008; Revenson & DeLongis, 2011; Chapter 3). The caregiver and the care recipient do not exist in isolation, whether a researcher chooses studying the care provider, the care recipient, or the dyad. For example, even if one focuses on the caregiver, characteristics of the care recipient context (e.g., limitations, needs, coping behavior) and the illness context, as described above cannot be ignored. As described in Chapter 3, there is much to be gained if caregiving were to be studied at a dyadic level. Congruent with the dyadic perspective, caregiving cannot be understood in full nor policy solutions be found by studying only individuals and, more importantly, only one level of analysis.

A biopsychosocial perspective

The framework sits firmly within the biopsychosocial model that is the hallmark of health psychology (Engel, 1977). Although biology, culture, personality, and life stage can be direct influences on any variable in the framework, they also operate as moderators of the caregiving process (Laudenslager, 2014).

Underlying principles and organization of the volume

Several principles and assumptions underlie our framework and guide the shape of the volume. Each of these principles is reviewed in at least one of the book's chapters:

1. *Caregiving is a dynamic and multifaceted process.* Although it appears quite easy to assess caregiver stress and caregiver burden with self-reports, there are many variables that combine to make that appraisal. Chapter 2 focuses on how caregiving stress affects mental, physical, and social health. Chapters 4 and 7, respectively, focus on two factors, *emotions and personality*, which can be determinants of caregiver stress and burden, outcomes of coping with that caregiver stress, and moderators of the relation between stress and health outcomes.
2. *Caregiving is a dyadic social interaction* that includes both the care recipient's and care provider's perspectives. Chapter 3 focuses on how caregiver research could benefit from a dyadic perspective.
3. *Caregiving is a dynamic process that occurs in a temporal context.* Caregiving changes constantly and over time, in response to the patient's medical and emotional needs *and* the caregivers' abilities, health, and perspectives on the situation. This principle is illustrated in all chapters.
4. *Caregiving occurs in a sociocultural context.* Chapter 5 focuses on gender and gender roles as women bear the brunt of caregiving. Chapter 6 focuses on both macro- and micro-cultural variables to illustrate how cultural values and motivations place boundaries on what is and isn't effective coping with caregiver stress.
5. *There is a need for care for the caregiver.* The final chapter (Chapter 8) describes short- and long-term interventions that are evidence-based, that is, developed using the scientific findings on caregiving. As you will read if you stay with the book, there is no simple solution for caregiver stress. We will need to look at individual-, dyadic- and social levels of analysis in order to develop the strongest network of formal services for the informal caregiver.

Conclusion

Caregivers are essential partners in care and will become the most critical part of the global health care landscape in this century. The unpaid care provided by caregivers represents considerable economic value to the health care system (Feinberg, Reinhard, Houser, & Choula, 2011; Rhee, Degenholtz, Lo Sasso, & Emanuel, 2009). Feinberg et al. (2011) estimated the economic value of family caregiving in the United States at $450 billion in 2009; this estimate was based on 42.1 million caregivers providing an average of 18.4 hours of care per week to care recipients age 18 or older, at an average value of $11.16 per hour. Outside of purely economic terms, this level of caregiving involves significant personal, professional, and financial sacrifices. As a consequence, it is important to understand those factors that affect caregiver's well-being in an effort to develop evidenced-based caregiver interventions.

2
Caregiving Outcomes

Revenson, Tracey A., Konstadina Griva, Aleksandra Luszczynska, Val Morrison, Efharis Panagopoulou, Noa Vilchinsky, and Mariët Hagedoorn. *Caregiving in the Illness Context*. Basingstoke: Palgrave Macmillan, 2016. DOI: 10.1057/9781137558985.0005.

There has been a burgeoning interest in caregiving with multiple reviews and meta-analyses having been published over the past 20 years (e.g., Li, & Loke, 2013b; Pinquart & Sörensen, 2003, 2007). Although the caregiving role is usually undertaken willingly and many caregivers find the caregiving experience rewarding and manage to cope with the stress and practical demands, it is often at the expense of their own health and well-being. Caregivers are appropriately called the "invisible second" or "hidden" patients (Brodaty & Donkin, 2009) with "hidden morbidities" (Braun, Mikulincer, Rydall, Walsh, & Rodin, 2007).

This chapter focuses on the outcomes of caregiving – how does caregiving affect the caregiver and in what domains? Numerous interrelated outcomes have been explored, including caregiver burden and physical and mental health indicators assessed across a wide range of health contexts (e.g., Schulz, Boerner, Shear, Zhang, & Gitlin, 2006). We provide a selective overview of the key outcomes of caregiving and the measures that have been widely used in the literature.

Psychological outcomes in caregivers and patients are intimately linked. Caregivers' health and well-being often deteriorates as the burden and stress of caregiving increases. Strain in family life, described as lack of support and intimacy or increased tension, has also been documented (Berge, Patterson, & Rueter, 2006). This distress, in turn, can affect the quality of care provided, putting the patient at increased risk of hospitalization or institutionalization which, in turn, can lead to higher health care costs (Family Caregiver Alliance, 2006; Yaffe et al., 2002). High caregiver burden may affect judgments of the medical situation as well, such as medical decision-making (Higginson & Gao, 2008; Sands, Ferreira, Stewart, Brod, & Yaffe, 2004).

The impact of caregiver burden on the caregiver

General considerations

Caregiver burden refers to the overall impact of physical, psychological, social, and financial demands of caregiving. It can be categorized as either objectively or subjectively. *Objective care-related burden* refers to indicators that measure the magnitude or intensity of the care task. This may be the amount of time that one spends on providing care (e.g., six hours a day or four days a week) or the particular tasks that are part of caregiving (e.g., maintaining finances, helping the patient get to medical appointments). *Subjective care-related burden* refers to personal perceptions of care – how stressful it is.

Often this perception is based on the balance between the objective burden of care task and the support that the caregiver receives in doing that task and the personal and social resources she or he has. As a result of varying resources, caregivers in objectively similar situations may report varying levels of burden (Lyons, Cauley, & Fredman, 2015). Thus, reports of caregiving burden based on caregivers' time input do not necessarily match the strain felt by caregivers themselves (Van Exel, Brouwer, Van den Berg, Koopmanschap, & Van den Bos, 2004). Low levels or relatively stable levels of subjective burden over time are typically reported in the context of medical procedures for which recovery is expected (e.g., organ transplantation surgery; Halm, Treat-Jacobson, Lindquist, & Savik, 2007) or illnesses that require lower levels of care. In contrast, typically high levels of subjective burden are found among caregivers facing conditions that have a progressive downward trajectory or high levels of dependency, for example Parkinson's disease or dementia (Etters, Goodall, & Harrison, 2008) or with a more unpredictable or variable illness trajectory (e.g., heart failure, rheumatoid arthritis, cancer). Moreover, caregiver burden may fluctuate over the illness trajectory – at diagnosis, during flare-ups, or at the end of life (Given, Sherwood, & Given, 2011; Stromberg & Luttik, 2015). This creates situations of changing demands on caregivers that create additional stress.

The time frame of care may also explain variability in caregiver stress. The burden of caring for someone with dementia, for example, may be different from that for someone with advanced cancer; in both cases caregiving may be intensive, requiring many hours of care per day, but in the latter case it may be for a shorter period. Burden typically increases in conditions when caregiving extends over a prolonged time (Gaynor, 1990) or when disease moves into the terminal stage (Grunfeld et al., 2004).

The concept of *activity restriction* is useful as well. Activity restriction entails disruption or interference with participation in valued activities and interests or conflict of roles because of providing care. Often caregivers are forced to put aside their own needs and activities, in the present and for the future. Social activities may be reduced and caregiving may create changes in employment (e.g., moving from full-time to part-time) or even withdrawal from the paid workforce. In addition to the added financial strains through loss of earnings (Whittingham, Barnes, & Gardiner, 2013), reduced contact with friends, family, or work colleagues magnifies the burden of caring. Caregivers describe feeling isolated and having no one to share their concerns with and express reluctance about leaving the patient alone to pursue their own social interests.

For many caregivers, the intense and sometimes unrelenting demands force the caregiver to balance these responsibilities with competing roles and responsibilities, including regular household work, employment, and childcare. This may be of particular concern for younger, female caregivers who have small children at home. Thus, being a caregiver of an ill person can also create the sense of being "in the middle" of multiple roles (Brody, 1985), where role conflict leads to greater role strain and emotional distress (Piccinelli & Wilkinson, 2000).

Mental health outcomes

The negative mental health outcomes of caregiving are typically manifest as high levels of stress and mental fatigue or burnout, increased symptoms of anxiety and depression, and low life satisfaction (see reviews by Li & Loke, 2013a, b; Pottie, Burch, Montross, Thomas, & Irwin, 2014). Numerous studies have identified the negative effects of caregiving on emotional well-being. Increased caregiver distress has been documented across a wide range of chronic diseases (Covinsky et al., 2003; Pirraglia et al., 2005; Raune, Kuipers, & Bebbington, 2004; Rhee et al., 2008). Many studies find that psychological morbidity experienced by caregivers is equal or higher than that experienced by the care recipients (Badr, Carmack, Kashy, Cristofanilli, & Revenson, 2010; Badr, Gupta, Sikora, & Posner, 2014; Coristine, Crooks, Grunfeld, Stonebridge, & Christie, 2003; Pihl, Jacobsson, Fridlund, Strömberg, & Måtensson, 2005).

As disease is a dynamic process it seems logical that emotional distress also would be quite variable and linked to points in the illness trajectory and health changes. Consistent with this, emotional distress decreases following acute care, hospital discharge, and procedures such as surgery (Halm et al., 2007), whereby recovery or improvement is expected. In contrast, distress peaks during acute health crises and worsens over the course of progressive debilitating conditions. There is evidence of escalation in caregiver anxiety, depression, and psychological distress as the patient's health functional status declines and as the patient nears death (Li, 2005; Stajduhar et al., 2010). Transitions in caregiving status can also affect the caregiver's psychological well-being (Bond, Clark, & Davies, 2003). Those with high-intensity, continuous caregiving and those who transition from low- to high-intensity caregiving report the greatest stress and are more likely to relinquish the caregiver role (Lyons et al., 2015). Moreover, this pattern has been shown to be reciprocal: caregiver burden increases emotional distress and emotional distress intensifies caregiver burden (Chung, Moser, Lennie, & Rayens, 2009; Cousino & Hazen, 2013).

Emotional distress can also threaten caregivers' commitment to the role and sustainability of home care. When caregiving becomes unbearable, the outcome is often placement of the patient into formal care or institutions (FCA, 2006). Although institutionalization or respite care programs may serve as safety valve for some caregivers (see Chapter 8), such services may also be met with mixed reactions by the patient and other family members. Interestingly, hiring a paid caregiver or institutionalizing the patient may not have its intended effect of reducing stress and may increase symptoms of depression due to guilt, grief, or loss (Haines, Denehy, Skinner, Warrillow, & Berney, 2015). Caregivers, particularly those who feel obligated to take on the role, sometimes feel guilty for needing a short break from their caregiving routine (Walker et al., 2015).

It is important to recognize that while some burdens are lessened with placement of the care recipient in institutional care, others persist or may even increase (Schulz, Belle, Czaja, McGinnis, Stevens, & Zhang, 2004). These may include the need for frequent visits, new responsibilities such as coordinating and monitoring care, and worry about the adequacy of treatment and the financial costs, as well as guilt. Asian caregivers report particular distress when a patient must be institutionalized, as moving care away from home conflicts with traditional cultural expectations of familism and obligation (Kayser & Revenson, in press; Lord, Livingston, & Cooper, 2015). Likewise, the social-normative structure of spousal caregiving, where the caregiving role is assumed as part of the marital commitment, may explain why spouses find it difficult to limit their caregiving responsibilities without substantial guilt. The belief that "no one else can do the job" (Beisecker, Wright, Chrisman, & Ashworth, 1996) coupled with concerns about the ability of paid service providers to understand and provide for the needs of the recipient and the fear that the recipient would feel abandoned are commonly reported by dementia caregivers (Cotrell & Engel, 1999).

Physical health outcomes

Many caregivers suffer from poor health as a result of their caregiving responsibilities; some describe being pressed to the point of physical exhaustion (Pressler et al., 2009). Many caregivers of ill people may not be in the best health themselves, particularly if they are older. The combination of prolonged caregiving and its attendant physical demands and resultant distress, as well as limited opportunities for restorative behaviors, may increase caregivers' risk for health problems (Fredman et al., 2008; Schulz & Beach, 1999). Compared to non-caregivers caregivers exhibit greater cardiovascular reactivity (Vitaliano, Zhang, & Scanlan, 2003) and poorer immune response (Kiecolt-Glaser, Dura, Speicher, Trask, & Glaser, 1991; Laudenslager, 2014; Lutgendorf & Laudenslager, 2009).

Caregivers' commitment to patients often takes primacy over their own health concerns (Coristine et al., 2003), so their medical needs may go unattended or neglected. As described in Chapter 5, this occurs more frequently with women. In one study (Pressler et al., 2009) older caregivers reported frequently forgetting to take their own medications. Similarly, poorer diet, exercise, and sleep contribute to ill health. Many caregivers recognize in hindsight that they could have provided better care to their loved ones if they had taken better care of themselves (Hunstad & Svindseth, 2011).

Caregivers' referral to support services may be influenced more by reports of poor physical health than by psychological distress. In a study of formal support services for individuals with stroke and their informal caregivers (Simon Kumar & Kendrick, 2008) caregivers with poorer health ratings received more services in the first weeks following discharge. Psychological distress did not have a similar effect on service provision, although 37% of caregivers were identified as experiencing significant distress.

Positive outcomes of caregiving

Many individuals choose to provide care to loved ones and to continue providing care even when the burden of caring becomes evident. Whereas practical considerations (time availability, recipient's preference) are often cited as reasons for taking on the care of a person, equally pertinent are the positive aspects of caregiving process that are experienced simultaneously with the challenges (Mackenzie & Greenwood, 2012).

There is an increased recognition in the literature for the rewarding and meaningful experience of caregiving for the care provider (Li & Loke, 2013a; Roth, Fredman, & Haley, 2015). Caregivers may find a higher purpose in life or become aware of their inner strengths as a result of their caregiving role. They may feel closer to the care recipient and grateful for time spent together (Parveen & Morrison, 2012). Even in end of life care, feelings of satisfaction are reported to outweigh costs (Addington-Hall et al., 1992).

Despite the emphasis in the literature on negative consequences of caregiving, it seems as though focusing only on the negative aspects of informal caregiving provides an unbalanced view and minimizes the value of caregiving. Some caregivers have reported that their happiness would *decrease* if someone else took over their care tasks (Brouwer, Van Exel, Van den Berg, Van den Bos, & Koopmanschap, 2005). These positive experiences have been referred to as the transformative aspects of caregiving. Transformative caregiving can compensate for and, in some cases, buffer the negative effects of caregiving and contribute to psychological well-being (Pinquart & Sörensen, 2003). These positive aspects may also be linked to resilience, the ability to navigate and spring back from adversity (Lepore & Revenson, 2006).

Caregiving outcomes over time

A few longitudinal studies have examined change in caregivers' health and well-being over time, although the study designs vary in the length of follow-up. The study period is often one year or less, resulting in a fairly compressed analysis of the effects of long-term care.

Two opposing hypotheses underlie longitudinal studies of caregiver outcomes. The *wear and tear hypothesis*, similar to many stress models, suggests that the long-term strain of providing care will lead to increased distress or poorer health. The *adaptation hypothesis* suggests that after a spike in stress and burden at the beginning of caregiving, these negative effects wane over time as the caregiver adapts and is better able to manage multiple demands. Most of the studies support the adaptation hypothesis, especially when "objective" demands and psychosocial resources are controlled in the analyses (e.g., Gaugler, Kane, & Newcome, 2005; Salter, Zettler, Foley, & Teasell, 2010). Some studies, however, support the wear and tear hypothesis. For example, in a national survey of depressive symptoms among 1000+ US cancer caregivers, caregiver stress and psychosocial resources early in the illness were predictive of depressive symptoms three and five years and eight years later (Kim, Shaffer, Carver, & Cannady, 2014, 2015). Many caregivers who were still actively engaged in cancer caregiving five years after the diagnosis showed a significant increase in distress over those years. Interestingly, approximately 90% of family caregivers had ceased being caregiver by eight years, one-quarter because the patient had died.

This brings us to a methodological point that affects comparison across studies. Because of selective attrition, the composition of the longitudinal caregiver sample may change as studies progress and participants drop out. Caregivers who are lost to follow-up assessments have been shown to have more negative outcomes at the outset of the study (e.g., Gaugler et al., 2005). Caregivers who remain in multi-year studies are more likely to indicate stability or even decrease in burden and psychological distress, as dropouts may be too stressed to continue or may have exited prematurely from the caregiving role (Gaugler, Zarit, & Pearlin, 2003).

Measures of caregiver stress and burden

A variety of measures have been used to measure caregiver outcomes. An exhaustive review and critique is beyond the scope of this chapter. A review by Deeken, Taylor, Mangan, Yabroff, & Ingham (2003) is somewhat outdated, but provides excellent information on many scales. The selection of measures for any study depends on the specific aims of study and the theoretical framework used.

There are a number of validated instruments for measuring subjective burden in different caregiver populations. Table 2.1 provides a selective list of some of the more commonly used and well-validated caregiver-specific instruments. A few of the more frequently used measures are described below.

One of the earliest and still used instruments is the Zarit Burden Interview (Zarit, Reever, & Bach-Peterson, 1980). Originally developed for caregivers of older adults, particularly frail adults or adults with dementia, it conceptualized burden as unidimensional and measured the burden associated with functional or behavioral impairments and the home care situation (e.g., finances, relationship with care recipient). There are 18-, 22- and 29-item versions as well as a 12-item screening tool (see review by Deeken et al., 2003). A study by Hébert, Bravo, and Préville (2000) showed that scores on the Zarit Burden Inventory were

TABLE 2.1 *A selective list of validated instruments for measuring caregiver stress and caregiver burden*

General measures (not illness-specific)
- Zarit Burden Interview (Zarit, Reever, & Bach-Peterson, 1980)
- Caregiver Strain Index (Robinson, 1983); the expanded version (Al-Janabi, Frew, Brouwer, Rappange, & Van Exel, 2010) adds the positive aspects of caregiving
- Caregiver Reaction Assessment (Given et al., 1992)
- Bakas Caregiving Outcomes Scale (Bakas & Champion, 1999)
- Revised Caregiving Appraisal Scale (Lawton, Moss, Hoffman, & Perkinson, 2000)
- Family Caregiver Medication Administration Hassles Scale (Travis, Bernard, McAuley, Thornton, & Kole, 2003)
- Family Strain Questionnaire (Ferrario, Baiardi, & Zotti, 2004)
- Care-Related Quality of Life Instrument (Brouwer, Van Exel, Van Gorp, & Redekop, 2006)

Illness-specific measures
- Caregiver Quality of Life Index – Cancer (Weitzner, Jacobsen, Wagner, Friedland, & Cox, 1999)
- Lay Care-Giving for Adults Receiving Dialysis (Horsburgh, Laing, Beanlands, Meng, & Harwood, 2008)
- Caregiver Schizophrenia Quality of Life Questionnaire (Richieri et al., 2011)

not related to demographics such as age, gender, locale, language, living situation, marital status, or employment status, implying the measure is appropriate for use with a variety of caregiver populations.

Other frequently used multi-domain burden instruments assess multiple domains or levels of burden rather than treating burden as unidimensional. The Caregiver Strain Index (CSI; Robinson, 1983) is comprised of five domains to measures negative subjective care burden (employment, financial, physical, social, and time). Validity has been established in caregivers of people with cancer (Ugur & Fadiloglu, 2010), stroke (Blake, Lincoln, & Clarke, 2003), and dementia (Diwan, Hougham, & Sachs, 2004). An expanded version adds a subscale measuring the positive aspect of caregiving (Al-Janabi, Frew, Brouwer, Rappange, & Van Exel, 2010).

The Caregiver Reaction Assessment (Given et al., 1992) is a well-tested measure of both the positive and negative effects of caregiving in five domains (scheduling, patient health, finances, family support, and esteem). The instrument has been validated among caregivers of older persons (Malhotra, Chan, Malhotra, & Østbye, 2012) and cancer patients (Grov, Fosså, Tønnessen, & Dahl, 2006).

The Bakas caregiving outcomes scale (BCOS) (Bakas & Champion, 1999) and its revised version (Bakas, Champion, Perkins, Farran, & Williams 2006) measure perceived changes in social functioning, subjective well-being, and physical health specifically as a result of providing care. It can be administered as self-report or as an interview and has had psychometric testing, as described in Deeken et al. (2003).

Conclusion

Several key conclusions can be drawn from review of caregiver outcomes. First, the conceptualization of caregiver outcomes is evolving in the direction of greater clarity and sophistication, attending to the multiple aspects of caregiving. Second, convergent evidence across a variety of diseases and demographically diverse study cohorts highlights the detrimental effects of caregiving on both physical and mental health, although not every caregiver's health and well-being is affected negatively. Third, measures have been developed within theoretical frameworks of caregiving.

Continued attention to the range of factors that may account for the inter- /intra-individual variation is needed to specify more clearly the full range of intra- and extra-personal factors that may affect caregiver outcomes. Better understanding of these factors is essential for the development of interventions and programs of support for caregivers (see Chapter 8).

Finally, it is important that future research and practice does not frame caregiving solely as a stress process. Caregivers can derive utility, value, and personal benefits through providing care. Given that health care systems everywhere depend heavily on the efforts of caregivers, it is important to assist caregivers in need of support to accrue some of the benefits of informal care.

3
Caregiving as a Dyadic Process

Revenson, Tracey A., Konstadina Griva, Aleksandra Luszczynska, Val Morrison, Efharis Panagopoulou, Noa Vilchinsky, and Mariët Hagedoorn. *Caregiving in the Illness Context*. Basingstoke: Palgrave Macmillan, 2016.
DOI: 10.1057/9781137558985.0006.

Traditionally, the focus of the caregiving literature has been on the caregiver. Specifically, the caregiving situation is viewed as a potential stressor that might lead to negative outcomes in the caregiver, such as strain, burden, and depression. This concern for negative outcomes seems legitimate, as findings have indeed shown impaired physical and mental health (Hiel et al., 2015) and even a greater risk for mortality within a four-year follow-up period (Schulz & Beach, 1999) in caregivers compared to non-caregiving controls. (Chapter 2 provides a detailed discussion.) However, the caregiving situation inherently includes two persons, that is, a caregiver and a care recipient (Fletcher, Miaskowski, Given, & Schumacher, 2012; Lyons, Zarit, Sayer, & Whitlatch, 2002). A focus on the dyad instead of the individual (i.e., caregiver) provides the opportunity to address important questions that have been largely ignored in caregiving research. For example, the caregiving situation may cause strain to both members of the dyad, and the caregiving situation may influence the relationship between the caregiver and the recipient. Members of the caregiving dyad may have conflicting views about the need for care or how it should be provided, which may in turn affect their emotional and relational well-being. More knowledge about such issues has practical implications for interventions aimed to improve the outcomes of both caregivers and care recipients.

Strikingly, the literature on caregiving has, for the most part, remained separate from the literature on dyadic coping. This latter literature focuses on couples coping with chronic illness and examines mutual influences of the partners on each other. One reason for the lack of integration of the caregiving and dyadic coping literature is the controversy concerning the definition of caregiving, as described in Chapter 1. Studies in the field of dyadic coping tend not to label one partner as the "caregiver" as both partners are facing the stress of living with a chronic illness, and not all "healthy" spouses provide instrumental or personal care to the patient (though caregiving tasks or intensity of care are rarely assessed). One might question whether we should consider persons who provide emotional support or companionship to an ill significant other as caregivers, or whether we should reserve this label for persons who provide instrumental care for at least a certain number of hours per week. Yet, many of the issues in caregiver and dyadic coping studies are related and overlap.

This chapter argues that caregiving research may benefit from incorporating a dyadic perspective. Specifically, we will use findings from the dyadic coping literature to describe potential benefits of examining caregiving as a dyadic process. Next, a number of caregiving issues that need to be addressed at a dyadic level will be presented and illustrated with previous literature where possible. Finally, potential limitations to the dyadic approach in caregiving will be discussed.

Dyadic coping research

Dyadic coping research assumes that chronic illness poses a major stressor for both patients and their partners and that both members of the couple are involved in a mutual coping process. In line with this, the developmental–contextual model of couples coping with chronic illness proposed by Berg and Upchurch (2007) posits that patients' appraisals of the illness and coping behavior (including seeking or offering support) do not only influence their own adjustment to the disease, but also the adjustment of their intimate partner. Similarly, partners' appraisals of the illness and coping behavior are assumed to affect themselves as well as their ill partners. This process of mutual influence may change over time and is affected by the phase of the disease, the life phase of the couple, and the sociocultural (e.g., culture and gender) and proximal (e.g., marital quality and illness condition) context. Although the developmental–contextual framework has been developed for couples, it seems to be applicable to other caregiving dyads as well, for example adult-children and elderly parents.

Studies examining dyadic coping with illness have focused primarily on the exchange of social support, collaborative coping efforts, communication between partners and intimacy processes, mostly in the early phases of disease. In the next sections, we will present key findings and point out overlap with and opportunities for caregiving research.

Exchange of support and collaborative coping efforts

As indicated earlier, dyadic coping research usually does not label the healthy partner as the caregiver and, hence, considers both partners as providers as well as recipients of support. In line with this, studies have examined and demonstrated associations between support provided by one partner and the other partner's adjustment in terms of distress or marital satisfaction (Dagan et al., 2011; Hagedoorn, Dagan, et al., 2011; Traa, De Vries, Bodenmann, & Den Oudsten, 2015). For example, both newly diagnosed patients with colorectal cancer and their partners who perceived little control over life seemed to benefit from their spouses' support. That is, the more spousal support they perceived, the fewer depressive symptoms they reported over time (Dagan et al., 2011). One may wonder though whether this exchange of support might be more important in early rather than advanced phases of disease. In advanced phases, the roles of patients and partners may become less balanced. That is, as patients' physical or cognitive condition declines and their need for care increases, partners may need to take upon the caregiver role and patients may unwillingly become care recipients within their intimate relationship. As a consequence, the effect or benefit of spousal support for patients and partners may be different in this phase compared to the early phase of disease (cf. Dekel et al., 2014).

In general, couples are most satisfied when give-and-take within their relationship is equitable, that is, when their investments in the relationship are balanced by their benefits (VanYperen & Buunk, 1990; Walster & Berscheid, 1973). However, in the context of illness, partners seem to accept some inequity if the patient has many physical limitations and they understand that the patient is not able to provide support as usual (Kuijer, Buunk, & Ybema, 2001). Nevertheless, patients with cancer (in different phases) who felt that they received more support from their partners than they deserved or felt that they were unable to do their share in giving support to their partners (i.e., perceptions of underinvestment in the relationship) reported more depressive symptoms (Ybema, Kuijer, Buunk, DeJong, & Sanderman, 2001). Particularly patients may struggle with issues of independence and autonomy, and the help of the partner might underscore their problems and lack of competency. In line with this, in a diary study among couples coping with Multiple Sclerosis, receiving instrumental support without providing such support in return was associated with lower levels of self-esteem, not only for partners but also for patients (Kleiboer, Kuijer, Hox, Schreurs, & Bensing, 2006; cf. Douglass, 1997). Interestingly, patients reported better mood when they *provided* higher levels of emotional support, whereas partners reported better mood when they *received* more emotional support. Kleiboer et al. argued that providing emotional support may be particularly important for patients because it gives them the opportunity to show appreciation for the help and care they receive from their partners (and restore equity within the relationship). The findings for partners may suggest that they indeed perceive the emotional support provided by their ill partner as a sign of appreciation and love.

One way to avoid negative effects of one-directional instrumental support, such as low self-esteem, may be to engage in collaborative coping. This involves joint problem solving, and coordinating everyday demands and relaxing together. Collaborative coping may be found especially in couples who view the disease as a shared problem (Berg & Upchurch, 2007), or a "we-disease" (Kayser, Watson, & Andrade, 2007). A few studies have suggested potential beneficial effects of collaborative coping for both members of the couple, in different illness phases. For example, a large cohort study of women with newly diagnosed breast cancer and their husbands showed lower levels of distress and higher levels of relationship satisfaction over time in couples who used more collaborative coping (Rottmann et al., 2015). Similarly, in a diary study among couples facing prostate cancer, collaborative coping was associated with more positive same-day mood for both husbands and wives and less negative mood for wives (Berg et al., 2008). In the context of metastatic breast cancer, Badr, Carmack, Kashy, Cristofanilli, and Revenson (2010) also found that the use of more collaborative coping and less common negative dyadic coping (i.e., mutual avoidance and withdrawal) was beneficial for patients and partners in terms of greater dyadic adjustment, although not in terms of fewer depressive symptoms.

In sum, the benefit of provided and received support, and especially the balance between the two, may depend on the illness phase. Knowledge in later phases of the illness that are likely to be characterized by more instrumental and personal care needs is rather scarce. Similarly, more research is needed to examine whether collaborative coping may increase emotional and relational well-being in couples as well as other caregiving dyads in different phases of the illness.

Communication and intimacy processes

Communication is usually seen as a key element of dyadic coping. Specifically, open communication and emotional disclosure (or self-disclosure) are considered to be important for both patients' and partners' adjustment to the illness (see, for example, Boehmer & Clark, 2001). The general idea is that emotional disclosure facilitates the cognitive processing of illness-related thoughts and feelings and helps the individual to reach a state of emotional acceptance (e.g., Lepore, 2001). Furthermore, spousal responses to disclosures may provide opportunities for validation, reappraisal, and finding meaning in the illness experience. Emotional disclosure and spousal responsiveness to disclosures are expected to foster feelings of intimacy within couples. The interpersonal process model of intimacy suggests that, in turn, intimacy reduces distress in both members of the couple (Laurenceau, Barrett, & Pietromonaco, 1998; Manne & Badr, 2008).

In support of the interpersonal process model of intimacy, mutual constructive communication regarding cancer-related concerns has been found to be associated with higher levels of intimacy in couples dealing with prostate cancer (Badr & Taylor, 2009; Manne, Badr, Zaider, Nelson, & Kissane, 2010) and self-disclosure and partner responsiveness have been found to be associated with intimacy in breast cancer (Manne, Ostroff, Rini et al., 2004; Manne, Ostroff, Sherman et al., 2004; Manne, Siegel, Kashy, & Heckman, 2014). However, there is little empirical evidence to prove that emotional disclosure is beneficial to emotional well-being (Hagedoorn, Puterman et al., 2011). For example, although a couple's intervention encouraging emotional disclosure did show an effect on intimacy, it did not reduce distress (Porter et al., 2009). Also, studies in which disclosure was observed during actual conversations between patients and their partners did *not* show more disclosure to be associated with lower levels of distress (Hagedoorn, Puterman et al., 2011; Manne, Ostroff, Sherman et al., 2004). Instead, both members of the couples reported the highest levels of distress over time if the partner showed relatively many disclosures, while the patient made few disclosures (Hagedoorn, Puterman et al., 2011). Perhaps, partners tried to persuade the patient to disclose emotions and thoughts by disclosing their own feelings and concerns, which caused distress when they failed to be successful at this. Alternatively, they may have felt alone in dealing with the disease, as the patient was unable or unwilling to show emotions and concerns. At the same time, the disclosures of partners might have been perceived as burdensome by patients, potentially because their partners' concerns reminded the patient about their uncertain future. In line with this, more communication from the partner about the patient's disease was related to higher levels of hopelessness in patients (Kershaw et al., 2008). In a similar vein, a communication pattern in which one person is pressuring the other to talk about a cancer-related issue while the other partner is withdrawing from or avoiding the discussion was found to be associated with more distress over time in couples coping with head and neck or lung cancer (Manne, Badr, & Kashy, 2012; Manne et al., 2006).

Though emotional disclosure may not be associated with better well-being, hiding one's feelings or concerns (i.e., protective buffering or holding back) and social constraints that actively discourage one to talk about the illness experience may have detrimental effects (e.g., Langer, Brown, & Syrjala, 2009; Mallinger, Griggs, & Shields, 2006; Manne et al., 2007). Protective buffering, that is, hiding one's feelings or concerns, in order not to burden or upset the other partner further, has indeed been found to be associated with greater distress in patients and partners (Langer et al., 2009; Manne et al., 2007; Ussher & Perz, 2010; Vilchinsky et al., 2011). A study by Langer et al. (2009) is especially interesting as it was carried out in the context of hematopoietic stem cell transplantation, in which the partner is required to take upon an extensive caregiving role. The study showed that both patients' and their partners' protective buffering behavior was associated with the motivation to protect the other (and the self). However, these intentions seemed to backfire in that patients as well as partners showed worse mental well-being when they perceived their partners to engage in more protective buffering. In another study, women with breast cancer who felt that their family members or spouses discouraged them from talking about their experiences showed lower mental well-being (Mallinger et al., 2006; Pasipanodya et al., 2012). In contrast, patients with a high need for disclosure whose partners showed understanding and validation during a cancer-related conversation reported fewer depressive symptoms over time (Dagan et al., 2014).

Stating that emotional disclosure does not appear to be beneficial in terms of better emotional functioning is not to say that communication is not important. Couples or caregiver–patient dyads do need to discuss issues concerning, for example, treatment options and care needs, otherwise misconceptions arise easily that may result in inappropriate care. Furthermore, sharing personal thoughts, wishes, or emotions may become especially important in advanced disease or the end-of-life phase. One may want to speak about unresolved issues and need to talk about impending death. However, these issues are sensitive and may be difficult to discuss for both caregivers and patients. In line with this, one study in the context of late-stage lung cancer showed that lack of communication could be ascribed to mutual protection, the need felt to remain positive and the feeling that issues were too difficult to discuss (Zhang & Siminoff, 2003). For example, patients did not want to talk about treatment side effects because they feared that treatment would be stopped. Patients and families sometimes held different opinions about treatment options, which made discussing this issue difficult. Another issue was smoking behavior. Some families blamed the patients for their illness, and patients indicated to hide their smoking to avoid upsetting the family. The most difficult issue for both patients and family members to discuss was death and dying. More studies that examine communication difficulties and the effects of communication on both caregivers and patients are needed.

Like advanced disease, cognitive diseases such as dementia may introduce specific communication difficulties, as cognitive impairments may complicate communication to a great extent. Again studies including both caregivers and patients are scarce, but one interesting study examined the communication between women and their husbands with dementia who had been dealing with the disease for an average of three years (Braun, Mura, Peter-Wight, Hornung, & Scholz, 2010). The women spent a considerable amount of time on caregiving tasks (on average, 72 hours per week). The couples were asked to discuss and plan a future event together. Negative (e.g., hostility), neutral (e.g., problem discussion), and positive (e.g., humor) communicative behavior was coded. The results demonstrated that wives whose husbands showed more positive communication reported less depression and distress. Also positive reciprocal communication was associated with less depression and distress in wives, although not husbands. This study shows that aspects of communication other than talking about concerns may be crucial for well-being, especially in a context where patients have difficulties expressing themselves. Braun et al. (2010) suggested that it would be interesting to study whether a training for caregiver–patient dyads focused on positive communication techniques, such as smiling and affective touch, could be helpful not only in promoting caregivers' well-being, but also in facilitating their competencies in dealing with the patients' limitations in communication. Relatedly, some studies examining dyadic interventions (including communication enhancement) in the context of early dementia showed preliminary but promising effects with respect to mutual understanding and the relationship between caregivers and patients (Moon & Adams, 2013).

In sum, emotional disclosure seems to be important for intimacy, but it does not appear to have beneficial effects on emotional well-being in the context of illness. On the other hand, hiding worries and concerns for one's partner or discouraging one's partner to discuss concerns or emotions does not appear to be an adaptive strategy. Though it is conceivable that partners want to protect each other from further burden, communication about illness issues such as treatment options and care needs is necessary. More research on the effect of different aspects of communication on caregivers' and care recipients' outcomes is needed.

Caregiving issues that should be addressed at a dyadic level

Considering that providing care is the primary task of a caregiver, it is important to know the patients' needs. For example, do caregivers know what kind of help patients want and need with respect to activities of daily living or in terms of emotional support, and can caregivers evaluate the patients' quality of life and symptoms like pain and fatigue? A related issue is whether caregivers and patients have congruent perspectives on the caregiving situation and formal care, including specific treatments or palliative/hospice care.

Perspectives on patients' quality of life

Quite a few studies in different illness contexts (e.g., cancer, HIV/AIDS, stroke) have examined whether the caregiver can reliably assess the patients' quality of life or symptoms (so-called proxy ratings). In general, the findings show that approximately two-thirds of the dyads agree on the quality of life, symptoms, or distress in the patients (Hung, Pickard, Witt, & Lambert, 2007; Libert, Merckaert, Slachmuylder, & Razavi, 2013; Mitchell, Robinson, Wolff, & Knowlton, 2014; Sneeuw, Sprangers, & Aaronson, 2002). Dyads show more concordance if the condition of the patient is either rather good or very poor (Mitchell et al., 2014; Sneeuw et al., 1998). For example, the agreement is higher if the patients have either very few or many physical limitations, very few or severe symptoms, or show high levels of substance use. Also caregiver characteristics have been found to be associated with concordance within dyads, albeit the explained variance is rather low. Caregivers who score relatively high on distress or caregiving intensity appear to underestimate patients' quality of life and overestimate their symptoms (Hung et al., 2007; Sneeuw et al., 1998). Furthermore, caregivers and patients may value different aspects of life and functioning differently, leading to disagreement in quality of life ratings. To illustrate, caregivers reported lower quality of life ratings for patients with dementia when the patients showed more neuropsychiatric symptoms (apathy and irritability), while these symptoms were not related to patients' self-reports of quality of life (Hoe, Katona, Orrell, & Livingston, 2007). In a similar vein, caregivers and care recipients may have different views of the caregiving situation. For example, caregivers (spouses or adult-children) reported more caregiving difficulties (e.g., family tension and insufficient money to meet care needs) than did the elderly care recipients. This was especially true for caregivers who perceived high rather than low levels of strain in their relationship with the care recipient (Lyons et al., 2002).

In sum, asking caregivers to report on quality of life and symptoms of patients may be a good alternative especially if the health condition of the patients is severe and they are less able to report on these issues themselves. It is important to realize that the perceptions of caregivers and patients may differ and both present valuable information.

Perspectives on formal care

One area where caregivers and patients may have different needs, goals, or perspectives is treatment and formal care. To illustrate, in the context of chronic kidney disease, studies have examined the preference for home versus hospital dialysis among patients and their caregivers. A review of these studies concluded that patients and caregivers perceive that home dialysis offers important opportunities, such as more freedom and flexibility, greater well-being, and improved relationships. At the same time, there are also concerns and fear about home dialysis due to the confronting nature of the treatment and isolation from medical and social support (Walker et al., 2015). However, most studies have focused on either patients or caregivers (Walker et al., 2015). It would be important to know whether patients and their caregivers show agreement with respect to these issues.

This is most salient in the context of advanced illness or the end-of-life phase. Some patients may want to stop treatment, as they perceive quality of life as more important than survival time. Their caregivers, on the other hand, may fear the patients' death and want the patients to stay with them as long as possible. In line with this, one study showed that the percentage of family caregivers who preferred life-preserving treatments was higher than the percentage of patients with terminal cancer who preferred such treatments (Tang, Liu, Lai, Liu, & Chen, 2005). Another example: patients may hope to be able to stay at home for as long as possible, but there may be a limit to the objective burden their caregivers can cope with, perhaps making hospice care necessary. One study examined attitudes toward hospice/palliative care showing that 51% of caregivers preferred such care versus 38% of the patients with terminal cancer (An, Lee, Yun, & Heo, 2014). At a post-bereavement interview, 40% of the caregivers responded that they utilized hospice/palliative care facilities. Noteworthy, the caregivers' preferences for hospice/palliative care were significantly associated with actual utilization, while the patients' preferences were not. Different perspectives on care may become even more important in the situation where health care professionals need to rely on the caregiver as a spokesperson for the patient, for example if a patient has difficulties to communicate. To illustrate, Reamy et al. (2011) found that caregivers of patients with early dementia did not have an accurate picture of the patients' values regarding care, such as autonomy, burden on the family, control over care, family activities, and safety, which is worrisome since caregivers usually act as the surrogate decision maker when the disease progresses. In sum, information about congruency and differences in perceptions about treatment and care is crucial in order to help these dyads to cope with the demands of the disease.

Potential limitations and problems for future research

Are patients and caregivers in a vulnerable situation able to participate in research?

One might question whether dyadic research in the context of dementia is possible at all. The answer is "yes". Research indicates that patients with mild to moderate cognitive impairment are able to answer questions about their own care and preferences with high degree of accuracy and reliability, and they want to express their needs and views on the caregiving process (Hirschman, Joyce, James, Xie, & Karlawish, 2005; Menne & Whitlatch, 2007; Whitlatch, Feinberg, & Tucke, 2005). Furthermore, higher caregiver burden in caregivers of patients with dementia was not found to be associated with a lower willingness to participate in research (Cary, Rubright, Grill, & Karlawish, 2015). Of course there are still ethical issues, and for each study one will have to decide whether the importance of the research question justifies the burden put on the caregiver–patient dyads. The same is true for patients and caregivers in the end-of-life phase. Hickman, Cartwright, Nelson, and Knafl (2012) asked principal investigators of end-of-life studies (43, response rate 63%) about the decisions they made regarding ethical issues. They indicated a number of strategies that minimize ethical concerns in the course of recruiting, consenting, and conducting research with seriously ill patients and their family members. More precisely, investigators showed heightened sensitivity to the needs of the potential participants (i.e., showing compassion) by allowing extra time to solicit consent, gently building up to sensitive questions, developing backup protocols, careful attention to the use of language, and methodological flexibility. Possible effects of study participation were constantly monitored (i.e., showing vigilance), ensuring that the research did not interfere with clinical care. One issue that investigators may need to overcome is so-called gatekeeping, meaning that care professionals may be reluctant to identify a patient or caregiver as a potential participant if they feel that the person is too distressed or otherwise less able to participate. In short, dyadic research in the context of cognitive disease and in the end-of-life phase is possible, but it does require being sensitive, compassionate, and vigilant toward participants, and showing understanding toward care professionals who are involved in recruiting participants or conducting the study.

Can we recruit sufficient dyads for caregiving research?

Recruitment of dyads can be challenging. A review of studies among couples dealing with cancer showed that, on average, 58% of the eligible couples were willing to participate (Dagan & Hagedoorn, 2014). This seems an adequate rate, but it is noteworthy that the range of the response rates varied from as low as 25% to as high as 90%. Also, the response rate could be calculated for only 33 out of 83 studies included in the review. Studies in the context of end-of-life or complex care needs also face difficulties associated with enrollment and attrition. For example, in a study by Shields, Park, Ward, and Song (2010), the required sample size for a psychosocial intervention for African American patients with kidney disease and their caregivers could be reached only by inviting a larger group than expected, with intensive strategies and effort. Specifically, using a personal approach (i.e., a social worker invited patients and the research staff contacted caregivers with the consent of patients), 49% of the eligible dyads was willing to participate, after an average of 1.7 contacts with the patients and 4.5 contacts with the caregivers. Various strategies were used to sustain accrual during the study, including check-in calls, reminders of appointments, special-occasion cards (e.g., birthday cards), and $25 payments per assessment to support transportation to the clinic and to reimburse participants for their effort. Although a total of 16 contacts per dyad had been planned from enrollment to three-month data collection, 27 contacts were actually needed. In other words, a dyadic study requires considerable energy and resources to recruit and retain couples or caregiver–patient dyads, especially when the patient is seriously ill or in the end-of-life phase.

Who is the caregiver?

In elderly couples, it is not unlikely that both partners have health problems. For example, one study showed that 42% of 995 older couples (aged 57 years or older) reported that both the husband and the wife had one or more chronic illnesses (Hagedoorn et al., 2001). The question arises whether we can label one of the partners as the caregiver. It may be that they are each other's caregiver in that one is still able to do administrative tasks, while the other can do the groceries and cooking. Or it may be that they switch roles based on whose health problems are most salient at a specific time. In other words, in some dyads, especially spousal dyads, it may be important to take into account the caregiving tasks of both members.

Conclusion

This chapter argues that caregiving research would benefit from a dyadic perspective. Although the number of studies focusing on caregiver–patient dyads is increasing, the majority of caregiving studies is still focused only on the caregiver. Some issues examined in the dyadic coping literature that focuses on couples facing illness deserve further attention in contexts where the partner can clearly be identified as a caregiver (e.g., in the end-of-life phase or dementia) and in other caregiver–patient dyads (e.g., adult child-elderly parent). Such issues include the exchange of support and collaborative coping, intimacy processes and communication, and concordance in perceptions about the caregiving situation, treatment options, and other formal care. Usually, couples' studies do not assess caregiving intensity or tasks; it would be advisable to include such measures to aid comparison between dyadic studies appearing in the caregiver and couples research.

4
The Emotional Experience of Caregiving

Revenson, Tracey A., Konstadina Griva, Aleksandra Luszczynska, Val Morrison, Efharis Panagopoulou, Noa Vilchinsky, and Mariët Hagedoorn. *Caregiving in the Illness Context*. Basingstoke: Palgrave Macmillan, 2016.
DOI: 10.1057/9781137558985.0007.

For better or worse, emotions are intrinsic parts of the caregiving process (Pearlin & Skaff, 1995). Becoming a caregiver can happen gradually or unexpectedly, as a conscious choice or a forced obligation. In the process of adopting the caregiver role, both positive and negative emotions emerge and are expressed. This chapter will provide an overview of the emotional processes involved in caregiving at three levels: adopting the caregiving role (emotions as motivations), maintaining the caregiving role (emotions as coping mechanisms), and impact of the caregiving role on the caregiver's emotional well-being (emotions as outcomes). Both positive and negative emotional states will be discussed.

The emotions of caregiving

Caregivers often experience conflicting primary emotions such as love and anger, which can lead to the experience of secondary emotions such as shame or guilt. This may result from the caregivers' inability to successfully manage their negative emotions (Rae, 1998). In a study of caregivers of terminally ill patients (Bialon & Coke, 2012), caregivers often reported feelings of guilt related to the care recipient's suffering or because the caregiver felt inadequate in being unable to relieve that suffering. Other caregivers reported feelings of guilt because they could not successfully manage their anger and frustration.

Although some emotional reactions appear immediately, others develop gradually over time in response to changes in the care recipient, the illness, or the caregiving context (e.g., the amount of help available to the caregiver). Often, caregivers are reluctant to express negative emotions such as anger, guilt, and frustration in order to avoid being judged by others or becoming an additional stressor for the patient (Burridge, Winch & Clavarino, 2007; MacNeil et al., 2010; Shaw et al., 2003). Caregivers often hide their negative emotions to preserve a self-image of a "good" caregiver (Rae, 1998). These emotions affect both the caregivers' well-being and the care they extend toward the patient.

Emotions as motivations for caregiving

Most family members become caregivers without much advance notice. The extent to which the caregiving experience will interfere with their quality of life and affect their health and well-being depends among others on both the overt and latent motivations for adopting the caregiver role. However, evidence on the emotional motives underlying the adoption of the caregiver role is very limited.

Theoretical frameworks for caregiver motivations

Empathy-altruism hypothesis (Batson, 1991). Seeing another person in distress can elicit empathic responses. Batson (1991) distinguished two kinds of empathic responses, empathic distress and empathic concern. Empathic distress refers to an unpleasant and aversive affective state, which results from observing another person in distress. In this type of response, caregivers experience emotions such as anxiety, nervousness, and distress, which are unpleasant and upsetting. Although empathic distress motivates helping, caregivers offer their help in order to reduce their own distress; helping the person in need is only tangential to this primary outcome.

Empathic concern is characterized by positively toned emotions, such as warmth, tenderness, and soft-heartedness, directed at the affected person. This type of empathic response motivates helping, intended to increase or improve the well-being of the person in need; any rewards to the helper are incidental to the act of offering help. Thus, while empathic personal distress is typically believed to result in an "egoistic" motivation for helping (Penner et al., 2008), empathic concern results in helping motivated by an altruistic concern for the welfare of the person in distress (Batson, 1991).

Self-determination theory (Ryan & Deci, 2000). This theory distinguishes the motivation for acting in a continuum ranging from controlled to autonomous. External motivation, that is, acting based on external rewards and punishments, is the most controlled motivation. A second and also relatively controlled form is introjected motivation; although internally driven, behaviors are performed to attain ego enhancements such as pride or to avoid feeling guilty or anxious. In the most autonomous form of motivation, that is, integrated motivation, the person integrates the societal value of behaviors with other aspects of the self.

These three motives can be illustrated within the caregiving context (Kim, Carver, & Cannady, 2015). External motives can be illustrated by the situation in which individuals take on the caregiving role to avoid disapproval from their social group. The introjected motive might reflect caregiving when it is taken on in order to feel like a worthy person or to avoid feelings of guilt or shame. The integrated motive involves loving and respecting the care recipient as well as acknowledging that caregiving provides meaning and purpose in life.

Dimensions of motivation. Quinn, Clare, and Woods (2010) have suggested that rather than exploring specific reasons for caring, it is more useful to categorize motives under dimensions such as egoistic or altruistic, and intrinsic or extrinsic. Intrinsic motives for becoming a caregiver include emotional bonding and feelings of usefulness; both reflect some personal choice in the decision to provide care. Extrinsic motives for caregiving are related to a sense of obligation and responding to social expectations, which leave less room for personal choice (Romero-Moreno, Márquez-González, Losada, & López, 2011).

The relation of motivations to caregiver outcomes

Intrinsic motives lead to more positive outcomes than extrinsic motives. For example, intrinsic motives have been related to less rumination, a maladaptive coping strategy (Thomsen, Jørgensen, Mehlsen, & Zachariae, 2004), and lower emotional distress (Knight & Sayegh, 2010). Similarly, Kim et al. (2015) suggest that the more autonomous (or integrated) the motive, the easier it is for caregivers to adjust to their role. With regard to extrinsic motives, several studies reported an association between "obligation-based" motives and greater emotional distress, caregiver burden, and feelings of powerlessness (Gross & John, 2003; Lyonette & Yardley, 2003; Romero-Moreno et al., 2011). A systematic review conducted by Burridge et al. (2007) found that feelings of reluctance toward caregiving expressed by informal caregivers were associated with decreased caregiver-care recipient interpersonal relationships, compromised quality of care, and more likely institutionalization of the patient.

Different caregiving motives are not mutually incompatible, as some caregivers may report high scores on obligation motives for caring and, simultaneously, high scores on personal motives (Walker, Pratt, Shin, & Jones, 1990). A single study (Hsu & Shyu, 2003) had suggested that motives could change over the course of the caregiving process: At the beginning of care, motives were mainly obligation-based, but became progressively more intrinsic. This change in motives could herald a decrease in caregiver distress.

No studies to date have examined the role of latent interpersonal emotions as possible motives, for example, feelings of emotional retribution, regaining emotional balance in the relationship, and unexpected emotional dividends, in taking the decision to become a caregiver. For example, the shift in the decision-making process from the male to the female partner in a couple might be a positive development for some female caregivers who up to that time were in an inferior position regarding decision-making, compared to their spouses.

Emotions as coping strategies

The stress and coping perspective

Maintaining the caregiver role is a challenging task. Stress and coping theory (Lazarus & Folkman, 1984), one of the backbones of caregiving research (see Chapter 1), defines problem-focused strategies as those that aim to manage or eliminate the stressor and emotion-focused coping as strategies aimed at changing the meaning of what is happening, even if one does not actually change the stressful situation. Studies indicate that caregivers use a large variety of problem- and emotion-coping strategies. For example, in studies of cancer caregivers, the emotion-focused coping strategies of avoidance denial and wishful thinking (Papastavrou, Charalambous, & Tsangari, 2012), emotional expression, searching for the positive aspects of caregiving, and disengaging from stressful thoughts (Epiphaniou et al., 2012) were frequently used to cope with the stresses of caregiving. Male caregivers appear to use more problem-focused strategies than female caregivers, but they engage in emotion-focused coping equally often (Han et al., 2014; see Chapter 5 for a discussion of gender issues in caregiving).

Although cancer caregivers frequently use emotion-focused strategies, these strategies do not seem to be adaptive. For example, caregivers of cancer patients who used strategies, such as worrying and negative emotional expression (getting mad or nervous, taking tensions out on others), were more likely to experience their caring role as overwhelming and to experience feelings of role entrapment and emotional fatigue (Gaugler, Eppinger, King, Sandberg, & Regine, 2013). In contrast, problem-focused strategies, such as trying to set goals and break caregiving down into manageable steps, were related to lower levels of psychological distress (Gaugler et al., 2013). Similarly, caregivers of patients with dementia who used more wishful thinking showed more depressive symptoms, while those who used more problem-focused coping showed lower levels of depressive symptoms (Piercy et al., 2013; for a review, see

Kneebone & Martin, 2003). In caregivers of advanced chronic obstructive pulmonary disease, cognitive-emotional strategies (e.g., drawing on strong personal or religious beliefs) were associated with lower mental well-being (Figueiredo, Gabriel, Jácome & Marques, 2013).

The studies described above are cross-sectional so it is equally plausible that the negative emotional outcomes lead to the use of emotion-focused coping strategies. It is also important to note that coping is a dynamic process (Lazarus & Folkman, 1984) and changes over the course of caregiving. For example, in a cross-sectional study of cancer caregivers, family caregivers in the early years of caregiving reported more helpless approaches compared to later years of caregiving (Tokem, Ozcelik, & Cicik, 2015). This may suggest that caregivers adjust to their role and learn how best to deal with the situation. In a longitudinal study of caregivers of individuals with Alzheimer's disease, engaging in more problem-focused coping strategies and less emotion-focused coping strategies was associated with more anxiety one year later (Cooper, Katona, Orrell, & Livingston, 2008). One could imagine a curvilinear relationship: coping is difficult at the early points in the illness trajectory because the stressors are new and also in the later years if the illness becomes much worse. However, longitudinal research is needed to support that explanation.

The (lack of) regulation of emotions can have consequences, for caregivers themselves as well as the care recipients. For example, caregivers of Alzheimer patients who reported low emotional expressiveness were found to be at increased risk of high blood pressure (Shaw et al., 2003). Furthermore, when caregivers were not successful in regulating their anger, the care recipient received compromised care (Dooley, Shaffer, Lance, & Williamson, 2007). Similarly, anxiety and depression were predictors of potentially harmful behavior toward the care recipient, but only when the caregiver was also reporting feelings of anger (MacNeil et al., 2010).

A host of interventions aimed at coping skills have been developed to support caregivers in regulating their emotions and to decrease caregiver burden. To illustrate, in one intervention, caregivers of person with Alzheimer's disease were offered a video of coping training combined with telephone coaching focused on the skills that were taught in the video. Caregivers who received the intervention showed reduced distress (in psychological measures as well as biological stress markers) across a six-month follow-up period compared to caregivers in a wait-list control group (Williams et al., 2010). Similarly, in the context of cancer, caregivers of hospice patients appeared to benefit from a coping intervention delivered by a nurse. Caregivers who received the intervention showed higher levels of quality of life and lower burden in comparison to a care as usual control group and an active control group (McMillan et al., 2006). Surprisingly, there were no effects found regarding the use of coping strategies. More detail on evidence-based caregiver interventions can be found in Chapter 8.

Emotional labor

Another perspective on emotional processes as coping focuses on the concept of emotional labor. Emotional labor refers to the external emotional management caregivers need to engage in to successfully meet the demands of their role (Hochschild, 1983). It mostly focuses on how individuals manage the expression of their emotions rather than the internal process of emotion regulation. For example, in terms of caregiving, emotional labor refers to the additional burden associated with having to hide feelings of frustration, sadness, or anger from the recipients of caregiving, and not on how these feelings are being regulated internally. In a qualitative study of informal caregivers of Alzheimer patients, Rae (1998) described different types of emotional labor involved in caregiving. Engaging in emotional labor frequently occurred and, in a sense, managing emotions became a caregiving task in itself. The most frequent strategy participants utilized to manage feelings such as anger was to remind themselves that the disease, and not the patient, was to blame. The study findings suggest that emotional labor, and, in particular, the failure to manage feelings, significantly contributed to caregiver stress and emotional burden. Too often, emotional labor resulted in perceived feelings of inadequacy when caregivers failed to manage or hide their negative emotions. More recently, two observational studies involving female caregivers of elderly adults (Silverman, 2013, 2015) showed that caregivers progressively learned to manage their emotions in order to provide better care, for example, by using positive actions such as reassuring, smiling, touching, gazing, and joking during moments of obvious frustration or exhaustion.

Maintaining hope

A specific emotion that has been extensively studied within the caregiving context is the feeling of hope. Hope is conceptualized as a dynamic emotional experience associated with the desire for something positive to happen, for example, a good outcome in a medical procedure or test. It has been linked to feelings of trust and optimism. In a meta-synthesis of qualitative research involving family caregivers of individuals suffering from various chronic diseases, it was found that caregivers experiencing hope were able to recognize more possibilities in a challenging and uncertain situation and thus to identify more ways to cope (Duggleby et al., 2010). Moreover this finding occurred irrespective of the caregiver's age, relationship to the patient, or severity of the disease. This flexibility, in turn, was hypothesized to further strengthen their feelings of hope. Caregivers who were experiencing less hope were less likely to be optimistic about their ability to handle the tasks associated with their caregiving role, or seek social support, both strategies that enhance adaptation (see Chapter 7).

Emotions as outcomes

As described in detail in Chapter 2, most of the studies exploring the impact of caregiving focus on the negative outcomes associated with providing care. Compared to the general population, caregivers report worse physical and mental health, including increased levels of worry and depression and symptoms of burnout (Fianco et al., 2015; Neugaard, Andresen, McKune, & Jamoom, 2008; Vitaliano, Young, & Zhang, 2004). Aspects of the illness context, such as disease severity and the care recipient's behavior, influence the emotional state of the caregiver and their quality of care, sometimes increasing caregivers' feelings of guilt and powerlessness (Trail, Nelson, Van, Appel, & Lai, 2004). Caregiving also can lead to positive outcomes, such as emotional growth, satisfaction, increased sense of control, increased intimacy, and increased sense of meaning (Hudson, 2004). Clearly, emotions are a central aspect of caregiving.

A study by Hirst (2005) provides a compelling example. The study used the British Household Panel Survey data from 1991 to 2000 and tracked individuals as they entered and left caregiving, recording their distress levels at yearly intervals. The study revealed an association between intensity of caregiving per week and emotional distress. Caregivers engaging in caregiving for more than 20 hours per week were at twice the risk of emotional distress than non-caregivers. This effect was more prominent among women. Moreover, caregivers in the intense caregiving group reported a higher prevalence of emotional distress in the year prior to becoming a caregiver. This suggests that adopting the caregiving role may not be a discrete event and although most studies indicate that caregiving creates or increases emotional distress, the most distressed may have already been distressed when the caregiving process began. Is this a personality disposition that leads one to adapt to caregiving in particular ways, some of which may not be adaptive? In addition, the study revealed that, for the high distress group, distress seemed to increase over the first year of caregiving, and remained stable afterward, indicating an adjustment to the caregiving role.

Many factors affect caregivers' level of emotional distress, as detailed in other chapters in this book. Gender (Chapter 5), culture (Chapter 6), and personality (Chapter 7) are three central ones. Aspects of the caregiver-care recipient relationship also deserve mention. Research has shown that the expression of relationship-oriented emotions, such as compassion, guilt, sadness, and happiness, has a beneficial effect on the caregiver's well-being (Clark & Monin, 2006; Tiedens & Leach, 2004). Caregiving spouses whose (ill) partners reported greater willingness to express emotions reported less caregiving stress (Monin, Martire, Schulz, & Clark, 2009).

Emotional recovery and bereavement

An important factor when studying the emotional impact of caregiving is emotional recovery. In the study by Hirst (2005), described above, recovery from distress – the ability to return to the levels of emotional distress before the initiation of caregiving tasks – could take up to five years after the time caregiving ended. The more intense the caregiving experience had been, in terms of hours devoted to caregiving tasks, the more prolonged the recovery time. In a study of spousal caregivers of dementia patients, caregiver's mental health gradually improved following the patient's institutionalization; however, after the patient's death, caregivers experienced deterioration in their mental health (Bond, Clark, & Davies, 2003). The end of caregiving marked by the care recipient's death leads to bereavement; the end of caregiving because one can no longer carry out the caregiver role may create a different range of emotions, including relief, regret, and shame.

Several studies have shown that caregivers' distress during the caregiving period predicts post-bereavement adjustment (Boerner, Schulz &

Horowitz, 2004; Christakis & Iwashyna, 2003; Hebert, Dang & Schulz, 2006). Higher levels of burden, feeling exhausted and overloaded, and a greater lack of support and work-family conflict were related to increased distress during caregiving and negative post-bereavement outcomes. Emotional preparedness has been identified as a protective mechanism against grief. Caregivers who saw themselves as unprepared for the care recipient's death experienced increased depression, anxiety, and complicated grief symptoms after the death (Hebert et al., 2006).

Conclusion

This chapter described the emotional processes involved in caregiving from three different perspectives: emotions as motivations, emotions as coping strategies, and emotions as outcomes. Various emotions can influence the decision of a person to enter, tolerate, enjoy, and remain in a caregiving situation. Irrespective of whether these include more feelings of love or obligation, it is important for caregivers to recognize their emotional life. Understanding the different emotional demands associated with the different stages of the caregiving process will allow psychologists and other health professionals to develop interventions that enhance caregivers' emotional resilience. Focusing on the positive as well as the negative emotional aspects of the caregiving experience will provide a more comprehensive framework.

5
Gender and Caregiving: The Costs of Caregiving for Women

Revenson, Tracey A., Konstadina Griva, Aleksandra Luszczynska, Val Morrison, Efharis Panagopoulou, Noa Vilchinsky, and Mariët Hagedoorn. *Caregiving in the Illness Context*. Basingstoke: Palgrave Macmillan, 2016. DOI: 10.1057/9781137558985.0008.

It is short sighted to study caregiving in the illness context without considering gender. Historically, caring for ill family members was an expected role for women within the privacy of the family. Caregiving is still commonly perceived to be a part of "women's work" in societies throughout the world (Esplen, 2009). This perception persists despite more flexible sharing of household tasks by women and men in Westernized societies (Hook, 2010). However, it is not just a perception: 60% of caregivers are women (National Alliance for Caregiving & AARP, 2015). The average "composite" US caregiver is a 49-year-old woman, married and employed, caring for her 60-year-old mother who does not live with her (Feinberg, Reinhard, Houser, & Choula, 2011).

Caring for an ill family member affects everyone in many ways (see Chapter 2), but some of these seem unique to women. Early studies comparing women who were caring for an ill husband to women with a healthy husband found that wives whose husbands had a chronic illness were less satisfied with multiple aspects of their lives: They were less satisfied with their marriages, with the amount of time the couple spent together, and with the amount of attention and understanding they received from their husband (e.g., Hafstrom, & Schram, 1984). They also reported being less satisfied with their own role performance as a mother, if they had children, but surprisingly, *not* with their performance as a wife. These data suggest that women with ill husbands felt an obligation to take care of their spouses and a responsibility to keep the family and home intact, but at personal cost.

Across the literature, the findings are consistent: female caregivers report greater stress, depressive symptoms, and caregiver burden than male caregivers, even when other factors such as the type of illness or the caregiver's age are statistically controlled (e.g., Hagedoorn, Buunk, Kuijer, Wobbes, & Sanderman, 2000); however, the magnitude of these differences is small (Pinquart & Sörensen, 2006). A few illustrations:

- After a heart attack, men reduced their work activities and responsibilities and were generally nurtured by their wives (Michela, 1987). In contrast, women who had had a heart attack resumed household responsibilities more quickly, including taking care of other family members (Suls, Green, Rose, Lounsbury, & Gordon, 1997).
- In a sample of 113 couples in which one partner had rheumatoid arthritis (77% women), women had significantly higher scores

than men on measures of depressive symptoms, illness intrusion, and sexual dissatisfaction – whether they were the person with the disease or the caregiver (Revenson, Abraído-Lanza, Majerovitz, & Jordan, 2005).

▸ Female caregivers may spend as much as 50% more time providing care than male caregivers (Family Caregiver Alliance, 2015).

This chapter describes how the caregiving experience may be different for women and men and suggests a number of explanations for why this may be. A few caveats must be acknowledged up front. First, the evidence base for how gender influences caregiving of individuals with chronic illness is limited. Much of the research has focused on cancer, dementia, or elderly care recipients. Second, we know more about women who are caregivers than men. Part of this stems from the fact that women (wives, daughters, daughters-in-law, sisters, sisters-in-law) are more involved in providing care to an ill family member and, as a result, make up the majority of respondents in caregiver research. That is, the samples in most studies are predominantly or completely female, making gender comparisons difficult. Third, few caregiver studies include responses from both members of the caregiver dyad, although that trend is changing. As a result, it is difficult to discern whether the experience of caring for an ill family member differs between women and men and patients vs. caregivers (see Hagedoorn, Sanderman, Bolks, Tuinstra, & Coyne, 2008).

Gender differences in caregiver stress and caregiver burden

Although caregivers of both genders experience emotional distress, many studies suggest that emotional distress is more marked among women caregivers than men (e.g., Hagedoorn, Buunk, Kuijer et al., 2000; Miller & Cafasso, 1992; Moser, Künzler, Nussbeck, Bargetzi, & Znoj, 2013; Pinquart & Sörensen, 2006; van den Heuvel, de Witte, Schure, Sanderman, & Meyboom-de Jong, 2001; Yee & Schulz, 2000). Women are more likely to report stress or negative experiences in relation to caregiving whereas men are more likely to report positive experiences (e.g., Li, Mak, & Loke, 2013), although some of these findings depend on who the caregiver is in relation to the care recipient (Lin, Fee, & Wu, 2012) and upon cultural norms for care provision (Chapter 6; Friedemann &

Buckwalter, 2014). This is congruent with findings that show women express greater emotional sensitivity to marital distress (Kiecolt-Glaser & Newton, 2001), and worry about family members to such an extent that caregiving in the context of a loved one's illness may be detrimental to their physical health (Helgeson, 2012).

Some studies do not find gender differences, but this may reflect the point in the illness trajectory. In a longitudinal study of caregivers of colorectal cancer patients (77% female), no gender differences in depression were found at two, six or twelve months post-diagnoses (Kim, Carver, Rocha-Lima & Shaffer, 2013). Similarly, no gender differences emerged in a sample of mixed-site cancer caregivers (65% female) at two and five years post-diagnosis (Kim, Shaffer, Carver, & Cannady, 2014). Levels of depressive symptoms and caregiving stress were extremely low in the first study and moderate in the latter, which may reflect a reduction in the need for caregiving as initial treatment ends and one transitions to survivorship.

Some have questioned whether these gender differences are related to the caregiving situation or are broader gender differences that have nothing to do with caregiving (Vitaliano, Zhang, & Scanlan, 2003). As described above, there may be some gender bias in reporting caregiver stress and burden. Women express emotions more and for them, emotional expression and emotional processing are effective coping strategies (Stanton, Danoff-Burg, Cameron, & Ellis, 1994); in contrast, men are less likely to admit negative feelings (Baker, Robertson, & Connelly, 2010). Depression has often been found to be higher among women than men (e.g., Nolen-Hoeksema, 2001). Women also report lower subjective well-being and perceived physical health than men in general (Denton, Prus, & Walters, 2004) and as caregivers (Pinquart & Sörensen, 2006).

Putative explanations for gender differences in caregiver stress

Why do women experience greater caregiver stress, strain, and burden? Although this chapter focuses on gender, it is critical to remember that factors such as illness type, relationship quality, and culture influence the way in which gender shapes caregiver outcomes. Stress and coping models, described in Chapter 1, would suggest that gender differences in caregiver health and well-being might be explained by gender differences in cognitive appraisals and psychosocial resources. We turn to a few possible explanations for these gender differences.

Gender roles

Gender roles are a key component of intimate relationships. The traditional perspective is that women are socialized to be nurturers and caregivers. Because of their early experiences, women are socialized into caretaking roles in close relationships and are more responsive to the well-being of others (Gilligan, 1982; Taylor et al, 2000). Mirroring this, men's less-active involvement in family caregiving may be a result of deeply held gender norms about masculinity that create barriers for men to assume those roles (Calasanti & King, 2007; Esplen, 2009). Both women and men may choose to act differently than these role proscriptions, but more often than not they are responsible for reproducing the social norms.

Gender roles can be "expressed" in many ways that affect caregiver stress. For example, the role of caregiver may be more salient to the identities of women relative to men, or women may have higher expectations for the quality of the care they deliver (e.g., Miller & Cafasso, 1992). Women may not ask for help with caregiving because the loss of that role is too great a threat to self-esteem and well-being to abandon (Abraído-Lanza & Revenson, 2006). Whether they are the patient or the caregiver, women continue to focus on others and maintain their domestic roles, both of which can create added stress (Hagedoorn et al., 2008; Revenson et al., 2005). Men often tackle caregiving in ways that are congruent with traditional masculine norms, such as remaining strong, minimizing emotional distress and focusing on caregiving tasks as small achievements (Calasanti & King, 2007; Lopez, Copp, & Molassiotis, 2012). Taking action may allow men to preserve a sense of control and counter feelings of helplessness (Lethborg, Kissane, & Burns, 2003).

Amount of care

Women may report greater *subjective* caregiver stress and burden because they experience greater *objective* burden. Women provide longer hours of care and more hands-on personal care than men (Miller & Cafasso, 1992; Pinquart & Sörensen, 2006). In most societies, division of household labor is inherently gendered – certain tasks are the realm of women and others of men (Hook, 2010). Women do more household tasks that need to be done repeatedly (e.g., cooking, house cleaning) whereas men do more occasional tasks (e.g., car maintenance; household repairs).

One could hypothesize that when women are ill and men are the caregivers there would be a shift toward greater gender equity, with the male caregiver taking on some of the ill woman's household tasks, thus minimizing the care recipient's stress. Only partial support for this was found in a study of couples coping with rheumatoid arthritis (Revenson et al., 2005): Male caregivers (husbands) picked up some of the smaller tasks but the larger tasks of child care, laundry, and routine cleaning were just as often done by paid help or another unpaid family member. A different picture emerges for female caregivers. In addition to their own tasks, they picked up some of their husbands' tasks (taking out the garbage, small household repairs) although they did rely on outside help (either paid or from family members) for larger tasks (outside chores, car maintenance). Interestingly, ill women did not report decreasing any of their usual tasks, even those with greater difficulty doing those things because of the illness, whereas men did. It should be noted that many of the couples were middle-income and had the financial resources to afford paid help. The picture may be very different in families with fewer economic resources.

In a daily diary study of United States married couples over 50 in which one spouse had a chronic condition that limited daily activities, Freedman, Cornman, and Carr (2014) separated household activities into spousal care and household chores in order to examine gender differences in their relation to emotional well-being. Care activities were reported nearly three times more often among wives than husbands and chores twice as often. Contrary to their predictions that caregiving tasks would have a negative effect on well-being for women and a positive effect for men, they found no effects for men and that wives' happiness was higher when they provided care to a spouse with a disability compared with carrying out regular chores. In another study of caregivers for someone with a chronic disabling condition, long hours of caregiving provision were more stressful for husbands than for wives (Lin et al., 2012), perhaps because they were less used to it.

Thus, although there are gender differences in the amount and type of care provided, the act of caregiving itself does not seem to explain gender difference in caregiver distress. Women tend to stay at home to provide time-consuming care to one or more ill or disabled friends or family members, while men often shoulder the financial burden (Dettinger & Clarkberg, 2002). Women do more, but are often happy to provide care. We will pick up this theme again in later sections.

Employment Patterns and Caregiving. Men often remain employed when caregiving, but women may not. It is estimated that between 20% and 39% of female workers are also providing care to someone in their family (Family Caregiver Alliance, 2015; National Alliance for Caregiving, University of Pittsburgh Institute on Aging, & the MetLife Mature Market Institute, 2010). For these women, there are conflicting demands of work and caregiving. In one study (MetLife Mature Market Institute, National Alliance for Caregiving, & The National Center on Women and Aging, 1999), 33% of working women who were providing care decreased work hours; 29% passed up a job promotion, training, or assignment; 20% switched from full-time to part-time employment; 22% took a leave of absence; 16% quit their jobs; and 13% retired early. A large Canadian study including 23, 404 individuals showed that men and women who were intensively involved in caregiving (> 15 hours per week) were more likely to be fully retired before the age of 65 compared to their non-caregiving counterparts, with relative risk ratios of 2.93 and 2.04, respectively (Jacobs, Laporte, Van Houtven, & Coyte, 2014). Female high-intensity caregivers were also more likely to work part-time (1.84) or not doing paid work (1.99). Although employment may not preclude caregiving, it tends to reduce the amount of time one can spend on caregiving (Gerstel & Gallagher, 2001) and, potentially, the quality of care. On the other hand, there is also some indication that being full-time employed may buffer the negative association between caregiving and well-being in women, even after controlling for the number hours spent providing care per week (Hansen & Slagsvold, 2015). Perhaps, paid work offers respite or distraction from caregiving or offers social and psychological resources to deal with the caregiving task.

Motivations for caregiving

Most scholarly research examines men's motivations for caregiving, while assuming it is a more "natural" role for women. Although it is counter to societal expectations of masculinity (Friedemann & Buckwalter, 2014), men choose to become family caregivers for many reasons, including obligations to family members and dissatisfaction with paid employment (Denby, Brinson, Cross, & Bowmer, 2014).

Although the number of men doing caregiving has increased (Baker et al., 2010; Fox & Brenner, 2012), caregiving by men *complements* women's caregiving and does not replace it. In fact men are often "pulled into" caregiving by the women in their family (Gerstel & Gallagher, 2001). In a qualitative study of breast cancer patients and their husbands, Zunkel (2003) reported that many husbands felt a responsibility to help with childcare, particularly when the woman was unable to do so because of side effects of chemotherapy or pain. Several of the husbands described this as "taking over things", which suggests that these tasks are still seen as the wife's responsibility. This is not a universal conclusion, however: in a study of diverse White and Latino caregivers (Friedemann & Buckwalter, 2014), male spouses scored higher on a measure of "obligation to care" and lower on a measure of burden compared to female spouses and adult children of both genders.

In a mixed methods study of 94 married couples, using a broad definition of caregiving, Gerstel and Gallagher (2001) found that women influence the amount of caregiving that men do for others; in fact, they refer to women as the "gatekeepers" for men's involvement in caregiving. Women who spend a lot of time caregiving for other family members have husbands who give more care. Caregiving husbands are not substituting for their wives, but complementing their care, so that the care recipient receives more care overall. This is congruent with notions of dyadic coping (Chapter 3), where couples view the disease as a "we-disease"; in fact, the male caregivers in Gerstel and Gallagher's study tended to use the pronoun "we" more often than "I" when talking about providing care.

Men are more likely to be praised than women for carrying out caregiving tasks (Harris, 2002, as cited in Lin et al., 2012). This may be because often they turn caregiving into "work", as problems to be solved (Friedemann & Buckwalter, 2014). One study of spousal cancer caregivers found that men reported greater self-esteem from caregiving than women, which led to less distress; this pattern was interrupted only if the women were low functioning (Kim, Loscalzo, Wellisch, & Spillers, 2006).

The gender difference in perceptions of caregiver stress is a product of gender role orientations and expectations. For example, Friedemann and Buckwalter (2014) found that men reported less caregiving burden than women in a sample of predominantly Latino and Caribbean caregivers of frail older relatives. This may be a gender difference, or it may reflect cultural gender norms (see Chapter 6). The Latina/Caribbean women believe that caregiving was a female duty whereas the men, who experience societal or cultural pressure to uphold masculinity, transformed the meaning of caregiving into a work situation. By doing so they could reframe caregiving as an achievement and feel proud of it.

Women's greater focus on interpersonal relationships

Although women's focus on interpersonal relationships brings benefits, it can also create additional stress for caregivers. Female caregivers are more emotionally connected to the family members they are caring for (Beeber & Zimmerman, 2012; Friedemann & Buckwalter, 2014) and, even if not reporting burden, are more emotionally affected by caregiving (Savundranayagam, Montgomery, & Kosloski, 2011) and tend to take on family members' burdens as their own more than men (Moen, Robison, & Dempster-McClain, 1995). Men are more likely to cope with caregiving by focusing on tasks and blocking emotions (Calasanti & King, 2007). We discuss this gender difference through the interlacing of several interwoven psychosocial resources: the personality traits of agency and communion; identity; and social support.

Unmitigated communion. Although the influence of personality on caregiving stress is addressed in depth in Chapter 7, the gender-linked personality orientations of *agency* and *communion,* and their extreme forms, *unmitigated agency* and *unmitigated communion* (Helgeson, 1994) have particular relevance to understanding gender differences in caregiving stress. Individuals with an agentic orientation focus more on themselves and use more instrumental strategies to cope with stress. *Unmitigated* agency involves an orientation toward oneself without regard for others and difficulty expressing emotions. Individuals with a more communal orientation focus on others' needs and interpersonal relationships, and are more emotionally expressive. *Unmitigated* communion refers to an extreme orientation toward others, in which individuals become over-involved with others to the detriment of their own wellbeing. These traits have not been studied specifically with caregivers, but may be important personality dispositions that affect appraisals of caregiver stress and burden.

Unmitigated agency has been related to greater difficulty in expressing emotions, and holding back is related to poorer adjustment among couples coping with cancer (e.g., Helgeson & Lepore, 2004; Mallinger, Griggs, & Shields, 2006; Porter, Keefe, Hurwitz, & Faber, 2005). Thus, caregivers who take it upon themselves to solve every problem and do all the tasks themselves may be more stressed, exhausted, and hopeless. Although unmitigated agency was conceptualized as a male trait, and indeed, men score more highly on this trait (Helgeson, 1994, 2012), it could also apply to female caregivers who feel a greater responsibility for the caregiving role and feel that no one else can "do it as well".

Unmitigated communion, a female-gender-related trait has been associated with poor health behavior, negative social interactions, and greater depression and symptoms for women who have had a heart attack (Fritz, 2000), women with breast cancer (Helgeson, 2003), and women with rheumatoid arthritis (Trudeau, Danoff-Burg, Revenson, & Paget, 2003). Individuals characterized by unmitigated communion are thought to be most vulnerable to distress in situations that involve caregiving (Helgeson & Fritz, 1998). If women score higher on measures of unmitigated communion, they are likely to see their caretaking responsibilities as the most important part of their lives and fail to care for themselves, socialize, and so on. This could lead to exhaustion, loneliness, and depression. Moreover, caregivers characterized by high levels of unmitigated communion are likely to engage in caregiving to feel better about themselves. That is, unmitigated communion has been found to be associated with an externalized self-evaluation (Helgeson & Fritz, 1998); individuals who possess this characteristic are motivated to help others to obtain the praise of others so that they can feel good about themselves. Such motives make people vulnerable to distress (Jin, Van Yperen, Sanderman, & Hagedoorn, 2010).

Identity. As described earlier, women often perceive caregiving as an extension of their usual (nurturer) role. Caring for others is such a valued part of one's female identity that it can't be lost or shared (Abraído-Lanza & Revenson, 2006). As a result, being a good caregiver may be more important for women than men. Women would then be expected to report distress if they feel that they have failed at providing care or feel as if they are failing the person. In line with this, it has been found that women who felt they had failed in their caregiving task reported more depressive symptoms than women who felt rather competent in caregiving, while this association was not found for men (Hagedoorn, Sanderman, Buunk, & Wobbes, 2002).

Social support and emotional disclosure. Another explanation for why women and men experience different levels of caregiver distress and burden has to do with another psychosocial resource: social support.

Social support has been related to lower levels of depressive symptoms among caregivers (e.g., Nijboer, Tempelaar, Triemstra, van den Bos, & Sanderman, 2001) and more positive emotions (Raschick & Ingersoll-Dayton, 2004). Lacking help with caregiving tasks also is related to greater depression (Mui, 1995).

Drawing strength from interpersonal relationships and relying on them for practical support are essential components of women's coping processes (Helgeson, 2012). Taylor and colleagues (2000) proposed a "tend-and-befriend" model to characterize stress responses that are more uniquely female. Drawing evidence from hundreds of studies of humans and other animals, they argued that adaptive responses to stress in females are likely to involve efforts to tend, that is, to nurture the self and others, and to befriend, that is, to create and maintain social networks in order to provide protection from external threats.

Women rely on their support networks more often; these interpersonal contacts serve as a place to express emotions, acquire feedback on coping choices, and obtain assistance with life tasks, such as childcare. Women are more likely to ask for support, use support, and not feel demeaned by it (Shumaker & Hill, 1991). Thus, coping through interpersonal means often confers benefits for women. At the same time, this mode of coping may result in additional stresses and poorer health (Helgeson, 2012) as women are often taking care of others while they are coping with their own stressors (and possibly their own illness), other family stressors, and possible work demands.

Despite the evidence that women have stronger social connections, they ask for less help with caregiving tasks than men (Friedemann & Buckwalter, 2014). It could be that, as described earlier, it is central to their identity and to ask for help is to admit failure.

Another reason why women may lessen their own requests for emotional support from the person they are caring for is the fear of increasing that person's stress. This reflects the coping strategy of "protective buffering", defined as "hiding one's concerns, denying one's worries, concealing discouraging information, preventing the patient from thinking about the cancer, and yielding in order to avoid disagreement" (Hagedoorn et al., 2000, p. 275). In a number of studies protective buffering has been found to make things worse for the caregiving spouse (Coyne & Smith, 1991; Kuijer et al., 2000; Suls et al., 1997).

Revenson et al. (2005) attributed some of the emotional distress of female caregivers to the perceived absence of spousal support. In a study of couples with rheumatoid arthritis, male spousal caregivers reported receiving more emotional and instrumental support from their (ill) partners and from their social networks than did wives of ill men. In contrast, wives of ill men reported receiving more problematic support (unfulfilled promises, criticism of coping choices) from their ill husbands than did husbands of ill wives. Revenson et al. also asked the caregivers about the support they provided to the patient; men did not provide comparable levels of support to their partners as women did. Moreover, female caregivers were less satisfied than male caregivers, female patients, or male patients with the instrumental and emotional support they received from their partner. However, there were no gender or gender-by-patient role differences in reported caregiver burden or marital satisfaction.

Taken together, it seems as part of what accounts for female caregivers' greater distress may be that they lack support from their partners, coupled with the physical and mental exhaustion of continuous support provision and the female identity of being a caregiver. One can imagine a scenario in which ill men reduce their stress level by focusing on themselves and less on supporting the caregivers, whereas female patients continue to care for their caregiving husbands despite their illness; this would be congruent with the personality traits of unmitigated agency and unmitigated communion.

Does the relationship of caregiver to patient matter?

We have focused on gender in this chapter, but in considering the influence of gender on caregiver stress, one also has to consider the influence of the caregiver's relationship to the patient. However, little research has explored how gender differences are shaped by the nature of the caregiver's relationship to the care recipient. When older adults need help, their spouses usually are the first to provide care (Lin et al., 2012). Adult children generally step in when spouses are not available. In either type of relationship, women are more likely than men to be caregivers. Can we separate the influence of gender from the influence of the nature of the caregiver-care recipient relationship? Is caregiving a different experience for female vs. male spouses than female vs. male children, for example?

Most of the literature looks at caring for parents, particularly elderly parents. Of the family caregivers who provide unpaid care to a family member of age 65 or older, nearly 80% are spouses or adult children (Wolff & Kasper, 2006). According to a national US survey (National

Alliance for Caregiving & AARP, 2015), the majority of caregivers provide care for a relative, with almost half (49%) caring for a parent or parent-in-law. A much smaller percentage (10%) cares for a spouse; however, those caring for a spouse or partner spend much more time providing care (21 or more hours of care per week). Consistent with the overall gender difference, daughters contribute a larger share of caregiving overall compared with sons, particularly the daily hands-on personal care (Friedemann & Buckwalter, 2014; Miller & Cafasso, 1992). Unmarried daughters often are (and are expected to be) the primary caregiver for frail elderly parents (Brody, Kleban, Hoffman, & Schoonover, 1988).

A meta-analysis of 168 studies (Pinquart & Sörensen, 2011) examined differences in depression and burden among caregiving spouses, adult children, and children-in-law. Spouse caregivers reported greater caregiver burden, and lower levels of psychological well-being (including greater depressive symptoms) than either type of adult child caregiver. This is partially explained by the fact that spousal caregivers provide more care and support to their ill partner as they are more likely to share a household. Gender interactions were not examined. However, these findings are tempered by the same factors that affect caregiver burden including the illness demands, illness trajectory, and personal resources.

In a study of cancer caregivers, adult children reported higher levels of guilt (specifically, inadequacy with regard to the care they were providing) than did spouses or other types of caregivers (Spillers, Wellisch, Kim, Matthews, & Baker, 2008). A study of family caregivers of older adult cancer patients found that sibling caregivers reported more burden than others (Chindaprasirt et al., 2014). In another study, spouse caregivers experienced the greatest burden and depression when their relationship identity included the caregiver role; adult children experienced the most burden and depression when the familial and caregiver roles equally comprised their relationship identity, creating role overload (Savundranayagam & Montgomery, 2013).

In a large US study of spouse or adult children caregivers of older adults with at least one functional limitation, adult child caregivers were more likely to report loss of privacy and less time for their family, social lives, and hobbies than spouse caregivers (Lin et al., 2012). Moreover, female spouse caregivers felt less good about themselves and appreciated life less than daughters. Comparing daughters and sons, daughters reported more negative experiences and fewer positive ones; however, they note that more of the daughters were ethnic minorities so that the additional stress may be a result of fewer resources. This study details how wife, husband, daughter, and son caregivers face different challenges while taking on the caregiver role.

Comparing male and female, spouse and adult child caregivers of older family members with dementia, Chappell, Dujela, and Smith (2014) found that wives emerge as the most vulnerable of the four groups when both burden and self-esteem were considered. Daughters experienced the highest burden but also the highest self-esteem, suggesting the role may be less salient for their self-identities or that the daughters derived self-esteem from the role. In some cultures it may be considered more admirable if you take care of your parent compared to taking care of your spouse ("in sickness or in health"). Similarly, male spouse caregivers were more likely than female caregivers or adult son caregivers to find positive meaning in care provision (Lin et al., 2012), perhaps because it is not expected or obligatory and seen as being more selfless.

Using a creative experimental strategy that asked participants to distribute caregiving tasks among a fictional family in which the mother had recently returned home from a hospitalization, Lawrence, Goodnow, Wood, and Karantzas (2002) found that when only gender was considered, the typical gender differences for adult children emerged: The two adult daughters in the fictional family were assigned more tasks than were the two sons. However, this finding was tempered by the presence of paid work and other commitments (e.g., child care); a child of either sex with other commitments was assigned fewer tasks, but this happened more with paid employment than with child care, which was seen as less of a competing responsibility. And, unmarried daughters were seen as having the fewest serious commitments and the one most likely to be assigned caregiving tasks.

Being a spouse caregiver is something of a double-edged sword: Most centrally, there is the possible loss of the most intimate relationship (e.g., Lopez et al., 2012). While writing this book, one of us (Mariët Hagedoorn) was reminded of a book written a few years back by a woman living with a seriously ill partner (Bosman, 2014). She left him when he became terminally ill because she could not bear being confronted with his life ending or the loss of that relationship. Although many in the media were quite cruel about her (seen as selfish) choice to walk away, many others understood her pain and her struggle.

It is important to note that the responsibility to provide care is strongly shaped by cultural values (see next chapter). For example, in a longitudinal study of Taiwanese family caregivers for stroke patients (Tsai, Yip, Tai, & Lou, 2015) there were equivalent numbers of sons and daughters identified as the family caregiver. In a study with a high proportion of Cuban immigrants to the United States, adult male children were the highest proportion of male caregiver (Friedemann & Buckwalter, 2014). The authors wondered if being single was a deciding factor for men to assume hands-on care or whether this was interwoven with the Latino values emphasizing the family; not being married does seem to be a critical factor for women as it presumes one has no family obligations "of their own" (Yates, Tennstedt, & Chang, 1999).

Future directions

Our understanding of how gender influences caregiving is nascent. Many studies include mainly or wholly female samples, which means that the experience of male caregivers – husbands, fathers, and sons – is not well understood (Denby et al., 2014). We know little about male caregivers – their motivations, emotions, and relationships (Lopez et al., 2012). Many studies focus solely or primarily on caregivers of frail elderly individuals or of people with cancer. Similarly, the literature on same-sex couples is sparse. As marriage equality became US law while this book was being written, there is a major gap in the literature as to how same-sex couples cope with other chronic diseases such as cancer, diabetes, and heart disease.

Gender seldom has been examined in conjunction with other contextual factors for their synergistic influences. For example, the literature on gender differences in mortality or morbidity rarely examines whether these gender differences are influenced by socioeconomic status. Yet the magnitude of socioeconomic gradients in health and mortality varies by gender; for example, cardiovascular mortality and morbidity exhibit a steeper gradient for women than for men (MacIntyre & Hunt, 1997). Both gender and caregiving place constraints on financial, educational, and occupational aspirations.

Conclusion

We would like to end on an optimistic note. Gender roles have changed over the past quarter century, which might suggest more flexibility for families coping with stress in the future. Men are taking on the caregiver role slightly more and women are less afraid to admit that they are not coping with stress and seek help. Women may report more distress than men because they spend more hours on caregiving tasks, because they are more open about sharing feelings, or because they feel it is their duty, as opposed to men, who derive more satisfaction and self-esteem from caregiving.

While not conclusive, research increasingly suggests that women caregivers report more caregiver stress, strain, and burden than men. However, this depends on the illness context (Revenson, 2003). We are left with unanswered questions; as others have stated before us, the relationship between gender, caregiving, and health is complex (Freedman et al., 2014; Pinquart & Sörensen, 2006, 2011). Given the number of women in the workforce and the aging of the population, it is time to find answers to those questions.

6
The Influence of Culture on Caregiving Cognitions and Motivations

Revenson, Tracey A., Konstadina Griva, Aleksandra Luszczynska, Val Morrison, Efharis Panagopoulou, Noa Vilchinsky, and Mariët Hagedoorn. *Caregiving in the Illness Context*. Basingstoke: Palgrave Macmillan, 2016. DOI: 10.1057/9781137558985.0009.

Much of what is written in the field of coping with health and illness adopts Westernized views of health, illness, and healthcare. Similarly, caregiving research is commonly underpinned by models of stress and coping, which inherently presume Western conceptualizations of family and support. Given the challenge of the global aging population and the diverse and growing ethnic mix of modern populations, this is unsatisfactory and creates a knowledge base that does not describe nor have relevance to all caregivers.

Globally, it is estimated that over a fifth of the population will be 60 or older by 2050 with geographical variations, for example, in China where the proportion of those over 60 is estimated to be one-third of the population (Liu, Guo, & Bern-Klug, 2013). These facts have clear implications for informal care provision in countries where families assume the primary responsibility. Although specifically addressing caregiving for an elder, Gupta and Pillai (2002) stated that, "families are more efficient in tailoring services to suit the individual needs of the elderly than service agencies. If cultural values and beliefs play a significant role in reducing perceived care giver burden, then it is crucial to provide support services to care givers and help them preserve their cultural beliefs and values during the period of elder caregiving" (p. 566). Pinquart and Sörensen's (2005) systematic review and meta-analysis of studies that compared White non-Hispanic caregivers with African American, Asian-American, Native American, and other ethnic minority caregivers reached a number of important conclusions. First, ethnic groups differed from White groups and from each other in ways that have serious implications for caregiver outcomes. Many of their findings are integrated in this chapter along with other evidence of cross- and within-culture variation in beliefs and values that affect caregiving.

Culture and ethnicity

We start with definitions in order to provide a synthesis of the research evidence and to enable comparisons between studies. Culture is reflected in what people say they do, what they actually do, and the beliefs that underpin the behavior (Hall, 1977, as cited in Gupta and Pillai, 2002, p. 567). "Culture" is an encompassing term generally defined as a group of people sharing a set of values, beliefs, and norms in their interactions within their environment. Culture can encompass the region or country of one's environment, as well as one's generation, gender, race (i.e., biological and physical features such as facial features, color), ethnicity, country of origin, language, and religion. All of these factors may vary within and affect culture. Although culture enables a community to function through a shared set of values based on common language, religion, and history, ethnicity itself does not predetermine culture (Kelleher & Hillier, 1996). Culture is also used to describe communities thought to share an identity and common language such as "deaf culture", "workplace culture", or "student culture"; these cultures are thought to differ from those inhabited by the hearing, those out of work, or non-students. Perhaps caregivers inhabit a culture that is very different from non-caregivers, and this shared culture may hold more influence on caregiving responses than that attributed to other factors such as language or ethnicity.

Ethnicity refers to the combination of one's race, for example, Black, White Caucasian, Asian (not technically a race but typically used as such) as well as one's ethnic origins beyond shared racial features, for example, Black Africans, Black Americans, British Caucasian, Chinese, Chinese-Singaporean, Hispanic. One's ethnic group may also confer a predisposition to certain illnesses due to shared genes of one's race combined with cultural influences on health behaviors, for example, the prevalence of diabetes among South Asians (Gujral, Pradeepa, Weber, Narayan, & Mohan, 2013).

People of many different races inhabit the same culture. For example, Black Americans and White Americans share an American culture although race and ethnic origin (Black 3rd-generation American, Black African immigrant living in America) may influence the extent to which a person feels valued within American culture. Smaller micro-cultures (e.g., South East Asian, Bangladeshi, Pakistani) exist within broad ethnic groupings (e.g., Asian), sometimes holding different religious affiliations (e.g., Sikh, Hindu, Muslim, Jewish, Buddhist, Christian – Catholic, Protestant).

Overall, culture, micro-cultures, ethnic origins, and religions encompass a set of consistent values and worldviews that shape behavior and actions. Thus, culture may influence caregiving behaviors by means of different expectations and social norms of support seeking and receiving behavior.

Macro-level cultural factors that influence caregiving

Collectivism vs. individualism

"Collectivism" and "individualism" are accepted terms used to describe the general orientation of those living within a certain culture, which are thought to influence how one copes with stress (Chun, Moos, & Cronkite, 2006; Kuo, 2013). Within collectivist cultures, community or family work together for the well-being of all, with group or shared needs emphasized over an individual's personal needs or rights. In such cultures, meaning is found through connections with others and with one's community; action is motivated by the values of interdependence, interconnectedness, reciprocity, and group membership (Morrison & Bennett, 2012). In contrast, within individualistic cultures, the uniqueness and autonomy of members is emphasized. "*In*dependent selves" rather than "*inter*dependent selves" are promoted, with the result that individual needs and wants drive behavior (Morrison, Ager, & Willock, 1999).

Governmental policies

The extent to which informal care is relied upon varies from one country to another depending on their current national welfare system. Informal care roles may be influenced by the extent to which informal care is supported by the state through provision of welfare benefits. While there is often no choice, it would be hard for a low-income earner to stop working to provide care if there were no financial incentives (see Arksey & Moree, 2008, for a UK-Netherlands comparison).

Socioeconomic factors including educational attainment, income, and employment opportunities will influence an individual's ability to access private care for an ill family member. Pinquart and Sörensen (2005) note in their review that African Americans, Hispanics, and Native Americans are commonly found to be disproportionately presented in the lower educated and lower income strata of the labor market; thus, insurance coverage for home care services for an ill family member may not be included at all or only minimally. In other countries, such as the United Kingdom that have a National Health Service, which is free at the point of entry, such socioeconomic differences may be less critical and factors other than socioeconomic ones may influence healthcare access (e.g., language, cultural norms, illness beliefs). When one adds in the fact that those from minority ethnic groups are, in most cultures, often overrepresented at the lower end of the socioeconomic ladder, it can become difficult to disentangle the influences of socioeconomic factors, cultural factors, and psychosocial factors on caregiving outcomes.

Social expectancies of care

Most of the research in this field centers around several types of studies: those of multicultural US populations, in which Black Americans and Latino Americans (primarily) are contrasted with White Americans (Pinquart & Sörensen, 2005); Asian populations, mainly comparisons between Chinese and people living in Hong Kong (e.g., Liu et al., 2013); and UK populations, with comparisons between White-British (WB) and British South Asians which itself includes four main communities: Punjabi Sikh, Pakistani, Bangladeshi, and Gujarati Hindu (Katbamna, Ahmad, Bhakta, Baker, & Parjker, 2004; Parveen & Morrison 2009). These studies highlight cultural variations in expectations of who should take on the responsibility of providing care to a dependent family member.

Some of these expectations have legal status. For example, in Southeast Asia (e.g., China, Korea, Japan) the expectation of familial care for an elder is typically upheld by the constitution. In China, the one-child policy has meant if a parent needs long-term care because of chronic illness, the burden falls on that single adult child (Liu & Cai, 1997, as cited in Liu et al., 2013). South Asian care expectancies tend to fall on female family members (daughters first, then daughters-in-law; Parveen & Morrison, 2009). In other parts of Asia, filial obligation first extends to the eldest son, although if this son is not married, a patient's spouse will be expected to support the care role; Katbamna et al., 2004). With regard to Latino culture, "the family affair of caregiving is so deeply embedded in the Latino culture that there is no separate Spanish word for it" (Evans, Coon, & Belyea, 2014, p. 345).

In the EUROFAMCARE study of caregivers for an older dependent relative in 23 European countries (Mestheneous, Triantafillou, & the EUROFAMCARE group, 2005), the family's legal obligations to provide care consist of an obligation to provide financial support and "practical help", the boundaries of which are not clearly defined. This obligation is stronger in terms of the potential for enforcement for spouses than for adult children, but with increased divorce, civil partnerships, and stepchildren, more clarity is needed if legal obligations are to be upheld in non-spousal relationships. Spousal legal obligation exists in Austria, Hungary, France, and Spain, and financial and/or care obligations are legislated for adult children in Austria, Belgium, Bulgaria, France, Germany, Greece, Italy, Malta, Poland, Spain, Portugal, and Estonia. In contrast, the state or local authority have the legal responsibility for care in the Czech Republic, Denmark, Finland, Luxembourg, the Netherlands, Norway, Sweden, Israel, and the United Kingdom. However, in all cases where there is a legal obligation on the spouse or adult child, the state will take on responsibility if an inability to care on the part of spouse or adult child can be proven, usually through means of testing and/or geographical availability. However, how easily and willingly would someone say they are "unable" to care for an ill family member? In the United Kingdom, caregivers have been recognized in the Carers' (Equal Opportunities) Act (2004); as a result, the administration of a needs assessment is meant to be standard practice, but implementation is variable. We have no data on how many caregivers invisibly take on the role, as the national statistics are not necessarily comprehensive.

National statistics

National caregiving statistics are seldom broken down by ethnic group. For example, the Future of Healthcare in Europe report (The Economist Intelligence Unit Limited, 2011) estimates that 3–3.5 million people are providing care for a dependent relative in Italy; 2.4 million in the Netherlands, and 6 million are doing so in the United Kingdom. Why is this figure so large in the United Kingdom, where there is a national health service? One reason is that much of what is categorized as informal care is not medical care but social and emotional care, neither of which is addressed within the national health service. Variations among countries also exist in terms of what is defined as informal care.

Ethnic differences in the characteristics of caregivers are not presented in the Future of Healthcare in Europe report; however, within the United Kingdom, these data are reported by Carers UK (2014). Of the 6.5 million UK caregivers estimated in 2014, approximately 600,000 (9%) individuals were from Black, Asian, and other minority ethnic groups. However, it is likely that the number of ethnic minority caregivers is underrepresented in these estimates because of lack of access for individuals with low socioeconomic status or use of other unknown care services among these groups.

Core individual values and their influence on caregiver responses

Values such as kinship, filial obligation, or familism have been found to differ across cultures and ethnic groups within cultures (e.g., Dilworth-Anderson, Williams, & Gibson, 2002; Heller, 1976; Parveen & Morrison, 2009; Parveen, Morrison, & Robinson, 2011, 2013, 2014). Both the extent to which the family unit is central in the culture and feelings of loyalty and solidarity among family members are thought to be at the root of providing care (Ramos, 2004). Familism, defined as a "strong identification and attachment of individuals with their families (nuclear and extended) and strong feelings of loyalty, reciprocity and solidarity among members of the same family" (Sabogal, Marin, Otero-Sabogal, Marin, & Perez-Stable, 1987, pp. 397–398) may be present in members of individualistic cultures, but is thought to be stronger in more collectivist cultures. Related to this is the construct of filial responsibility or filial piety, which refers to the obligations of respecting, supporting, and taking care of older family members (Tang, 2006).

In a cross-sectional study (Parveen et al., 2013), British South Asian caregivers had higher levels of familism, used more behavioral disengagement and religious coping, and reported having less support than WB caregivers. The WB caregivers were more likely to cope with substance use or humor. In a longitudinal study with these groups (Parveen et al., 2014), coping strategies mediated the effects of familism on caregiver outcomes. Qualitative data suggest that British Bangladeshi, Pakistani, and Indian caregivers reported greater use of religious coping than WB caregivers. The South Asian caregivers accepted the caring role as one given to them by God; as a British-Bangladeshi female, age 39, caring for her daughter, stated, "However much we are doing, we have to do. God gave us them (the care recipient), 6 or 7 months ago it was hard but now I'm used to it" (Parveen et al., 2011, p. 868).

Acceptance of the caregiver role, or more explicitly, self-identification as a caregiver, varies. The extent to which the role is an "embraced: identity" rather than an "enforced", "absorbed", or "rejected" one is likely be influenced by both gender and culture, as both shape expectations placed upon caregivers (Hughes, Locock, & Ziebland, 2013). Although holding strong cultural norms of filial obligation has been hypothesized to mediate the negative effects of caregiving (Gupta & Pillai, 2002), research does not support this unequivocally. Among Asian Indian caregivers, caregiver burden was higher in those who endorsed high familism (Gupta, Rowe, & Pillai 2009), but this association was not replicated among Hispanic caregivers (Koerner & Shirai, 2012). Filial responsibility has been shown to be related to poorer self-rated health among White Canadian caregivers but to better health and lower burden among Chinese Canadian caregivers (Funk, Chappell, & Liu, 2013; Lai, 2010). This was attributed to different cultural meanings of filial responsibility – as burdensome among the former, but honorable in the latter (Funk et al., 2013).

Filial obligation in China requires adult children to fulfill their caregiving responsibility; this often necessitates co-residing with the ill parent or relative (Liu et al., 2013). Co-residency as a result of illness or increased care needs is also reported in studies of Indian, African American, Asian-American, Mexican, Hispanic, or Latino caregivers (Evans et al., 2014; Gupta & Pillai, 2002; Hays, Pieper, & Purser, 2003). The results of a systematic review contradict this: Ethnic minority caregivers were no more likely to live with the care recipient than were non-Hispanic White caregivers (Pinquart & Sörensen, 2005), although ethnic minority caregivers reported providing care for more hours a week. Generally, in non-Eastern cultures it is more likely that an adult child caregiver will live elsewhere, which may explain the often lower levels of caregiver burden in adult children compared to co-resident caregivers, usually spouses (Pinquart & Sörensen, 2007). Assumptions of extended families as the norm in Asian communities are being challenged by increasing Westernization, changes in gender roles, and growing preferences to have one's own home (Ahmad, 2000; Katbamna et al., 2004).

Micro-level cultural variations

Age

British South Asian caregivers are often found to be significantly younger than WB caregivers (Carers UK, 2001; Orbach, 2007; Parveen & Morrison, 2012) similar to many micro-cultures in the United States (e.g., Giunta, Chow, Scharlach, & Dal Santo, 2004). In a systematic review, caregivers in mixed ethnic minority groups were younger than non-Hispanic White caregivers (Pinquart & Sörensen, 2005). However, such age differences may reflect the fact that in many Western cultures,

Whites typically have a longer life expectancy than those in ethnic minority groups (Pinquart & Sörensen, 2005). Age differences also reflect cultural and ethnic variations in who takes on the caregiver role, the spouse or adult child, with the latter represented more frequently within ethnic minority caregiver samples.

Gender roles

As described in detail in the previous chapter, women take on caring roles more than men do, regardless of culture. This discrepancy is smaller within more individualistic and Western countries, as gender egalitarianism tends to be stronger (United Nations, 2003). It is interesting that this egalitarianism extends to Singapore, an Eastern country, however one with a significant Western influence (Li, Ngin, & Teo, 2008).

Gender also influences the type of care task performed. Some of the tasks typically carried out by males may not be considered as caregiving in certain cultures. For example, fathers of a child with a disability may make structural adaptations to the home or complete paperwork to access welfare benefit. Although some may not consider these as caregiving, such tasks underpin the ability of the mother to provide daily care (Katbamna et al., 2004). Further complexities exist where there are moral or religious codes of conduct to consider. For example, a Muslim female may not have physical contact with any adult male other than her husband, making it difficult for daughters-in-law or sisters to help care for fathers, brothers, or male in-laws.

Cultural variations in perceptions of illness

There is considerable evidence of variation in perceptions of illness and disability and in expectancies for treatment and caregiving both within and across cultures. For example, the dialectical belief systems that commonly exist in collectivist East Asian cultures support the principles of *contradiction, change, and holism*. Contradiction is when two opposing propositions can be true at the same time, for example, the fact that that negative and positive aspects of caring may coexist. The principle of change supposes that it is normal for the universe and life to be unpredictable and changeable. With this belief, taking on the caregiver role due to a family member's sudden illness may have less psychological impact. The perspective of holism, that all things are interconnected (Spencer-Rodgers, Williams, & Peng, 2010), opposes the common

Western expectancies of life and illness as explainable and reducible to stated causes. Because of these beliefs, East Asian caregivers may accept caregiving as part of their role and life's plan for them to take on the role at this time and in this context.

Studies on Asian cultures, as well as some general population studies, have found that individuals consider the state of health as one reflecting balance between internal and external systems (Quah & Bishop 1996). Health is viewed as a harmonious state where the internal and external systems are in balance, for example yin and yang (Chinese) or hot and cold (Vietnamese). Traditional Chinese medicine and Ayurvedic medicine take this holistic view of health and illness, rather than addressing only the purely physical or observable aspects. A holistic view is thought to influence perceptions of giving and receiving support, which may help explain some of the cultural differences in caregiving motivations and experiences: beliefs about illness and treatment may shape a person's willingness to provide care (Hunt & Smith, 2004; Williams, Morrison, & Robinson, 2014).

Cultural differences are also seen in attributions of causes of illness or misfortune. For example, illness is commonly attributed to predestination within Eastern cultures, and more often to external causes, such as the will of God, among African Americans and Latinos than Whites (Vaughn, Jacquez, & Baker, 2009). Mexican Americans, who believe in two sources of illness – one natural, one supernatural, commonly believe that healing is a gift from God (Trotter, 2001).

There is some research evidence that the extent to which an individual adopts or adheres to the values of their ethnic group, that is the extent to which they embrace their cultural identity, influences attitudes toward health care and caregiving. In a rare study of North American Indian caregivers (Goins et al., 2011), a stronger cultural identity, as shown through use of Native language, greater involvement in Native events such as powwow or potlatches, and the use of traditional healing practices, was associated with a greater likelihood of providing care to a dependent family member.

Caregivers' health and illness beliefs influence their coping and caregiving behaviors. This would be congruent with both the self-regulation model (Leventhal et al., 2012) and the sociocultural stress-coping model (Knight & Sayegh, 2010). Few studies, however, have used these models in caregiving research. A study of kidney disease patients undergoing dialysis (Kim, Pavlish, Evangelista, Kopple, & Phillips, 2012) identified differences in treatment beliefs and personal control beliefs among African Americans, Hispanics, Korean-Americans and Filipino-Americans. African American patients reported less personal control over their illness and Korean patients reported higher emotional perceptions. One wonders if their caregivers would show similar differences and whether it affects caregiving responses and outcomes. Motivations and willingness to accept and maintain the caregiver role are likely to be shaped by illness beliefs that are themselves shaped by culture.

Motivation to provide care

Providing support to another can be considered a prosocial behavior, that is, an action characterized by love, empathy, trust, and altruism. Several studies have addressed the issue of motivations to care using the Motivations in Elder Caregiving Scale developed by Lyonette and Yardley (2003). This scale contains two subscales, one addressing intrinsic motivations to provide care (IMEC) and the other addressing extrinsic motivations to provide care (EMEC). Intrinsic motivations involve a desire to care, resistance to formal care and seeing caregiving as a part of one's identity; extrinsic motivations involve a sense of duty, lack of choice, guilt, or perceived disapproval from others for not providing care. The IMEC and EMEC subscales have been differentially associated with caregiver satisfaction (positively in those intrinsically motivated, negatively with those extrinsically motivated) and with caregiver stress (positively in those extrinsically motivated, and not associated with intrinsic motivations). Motivations to care may vary as a function of the nature of the care required, specifically, emotional or practical support vs. more intimate nursing care. (Chapter 4 discusses motivations to care in more detail.)

This is recognized in the Willingness to Care scale (Abell, 2001), which distinguishes between willingness to provide emotional care (comfort when the care recipient is sad), nursing care, and instrumental care (e.g., laundry). In a longitudinal study using this scale, Parveen and colleagues (2013) examined the relation of willingness to care with caregiver outcomes in two caregiver groups – WB and British South Asian (BSA). Although levels of willingness to care did not differ between the two cultural groups, willingness to provide instrumental and nursing care were associated with greater anxiety for the BSA caregivers but lower anxiety for the WB caregivers. Willingness to provide emotional care was unrelated to anxiety or depression among BSA caregivers but was associated with lower anxiety among WB caregivers.

A possible explanation for these findings are beliefs held by these micro-cultures. A focus group study exploring subgroup differences within a British South Asian sample (Parveen et al., 2011) found that British Bangladeshi, British Pakistani, and British Indian caregivers were more likely to report extrinsic motivations for care than their WB counterparts. For example, a British-Bangladeshi woman caring for her husband explained, "It is our duty towards our family, we wouldn't get anybody else to come and do it. We will have to do it. We won't hand our family over to anyone else, it's our blood. We'll do it ourselves. We will try as long as we are here. We don't want anybody else to look after our family" (p. 866). In contrast an older WB female stated, "It's your husband, you've been married to him a long time, it's in your marriage vows, it's something you want to do for him" (p. 866). However, being extrinsically (vs. intrinsically) motivated did not necessarily mean that these women were unwilling to perform the caregiving role. Even for those unwilling to care, an affiliation to cultural norms and a reluctance to share care with anyone outside the family was evident. There were a few instances in which daughters felt they had little choice but to provide care, often due to a failure on the part of the daughter-in-law to meet her responsibilities. In British South Asian culture, the eldest son's wife is expected to be first to take on care of her mother-in-law.

What is worth noting is the potential relevance of relationship quality to such findings. Relationship quality is a significant predictor itself of caregiver outcomes. Motivations to provide care combine with factors such as the care recipient's resistance to being cared for or respect for the care recipient to explain caregiver outcomes. More specifically, better relationship quality and intrinsic motivations to care were the strongest predictors of caregiver satisfaction in this study of female caregivers, whereas extrinsic motivations and poor relationship quality were the strongest predictors of caregiver stress (Lyonette & Yardley, 2003).

Cultural variations in caregivers' experience

Cultural variations exist in the willingness to discuss illness or family issues outside the family. For example, acknowledging the negative impact of caring may considered to be culturally inappropriate, which may bias findings (Coon et al., 2004; Gallagher-Thomson, Solano, Coon, & Areán, 2003). Few studies make use of non-caregiver comparison samples, so that one cannot conclude that levels of caregiver stress, burden, or positive outcomes are due to caregiving alone (Vitaliano, Zhang, & Scanlon, 2003). One exception is a recent study of Thai caregivers (Lawang, Horey, & Blackford, 2015) in which caregivers of a family member with an acquired physical disability (e.g., stroke or fall) reported poorer emotional and physical well-being than age matched non-caregivers.

Negative aspects of caregiving

Across many studies, ethnic minority caregivers experience less burden and depression than White caregivers (Pinquart & Sörensen, 2005). This is partially explained by who is doing the caregiving, as younger caregivers (adult children) more often provide care than spouses. However, differences in familism, coping, beliefs, and use of social support have independent or interacting effects on such caregiver outcomes.

Notions of familism, kinship ties, and collectivism have led to the assumption that ethnic minority caregivers have an extended familial social network that will provide more sources of support to the ill family member and to the caregiver (e.g., Aranda & Knight, 1997). Ethnic minority caregivers generally report higher informal social support than White non-Hispanic caregivers. However, differences emerge with regard to the use of formal support; for example, Asian-Americans accept less than all other caregiver groups (Pinquart & Sörensen, 2005) and Korean caregivers reported lower level of emotional and instrumental support than American caregivers (Youn, Knight, Jeong, & Benton, 1999). This echoes Giunta et al.'s (2004) findings that White and African American caregivers were two times more likely to use formal services than Asian Americans, Latino Americans, or those from Hawaii or the Pacific Islands. Many Asian cultures are bound by a norm of suppression of anger, although the relationship between emotional expression and caregiver acceptance of support remains unexplored. It has been suggested that familism may increase feelings of obligation and thereby account for increased perceived caregiver burden and distress (e.g., Parveen et al., 2013). However, two related studies conducted with resident Koreans, Korean-Americans, and Whites found inconsistent findings as to the relationship between familism and anxiety or depression (Chun, Knight, & Youn, 2007; Youn et al., 1999).

At the same time, studies have failed to confirm the assumption that Asian cultures receive greater familial or informal support. For example, British South Asian caregivers (Punjabi Sikh, Guajarati Hindu, Bangladeshi, and Pakistani caregivers) reported having limited support in both their nuclear and extended households (Katbamna et al., 2004) and significantly less support than WB caregivers (Parveen et al., 2013). Interestingly the finding of *less* support tends to emerge from qualitative studies using either interviews or focus group methods. Perhaps the expression of feelings of frustration at the lack of support and isolation in the caregiver role is more easily expressed with such methodologies. As Katbamna et al. (2004) conclude, the evidence, at least from South Asian communities, is that this ethnic minority "as a group are no more likely than caregivers from other communities to be assured of support from wider kinship and social networks" (p. 404). Avoiding making stereotypical judgments about familial support is important as otherwise we risk assuming that there is a lesser need for formal services to caregivers among particular micro-cultures.

Positive aspects of caregiving

In the multinational EUROFAMCARE study (Triantafillou et al., 2010), caregivers in the United Kingdom and Sweden reported the highest quality of life (65% and 67% respectively), whereas those in Greece and Italy reported the lowest (50% and 51%). This was tentatively attributed to national caregiver policies and, consequently, the greater availability of services in the United Kingdom and Sweden. In a longitudinal study of British caregivers, familism was associated with caregiver gains, including new skills and increased closeness to family (Parveen & Morrison, 2012). Familism was associated with greater caregiver satisfaction among Chinese caregivers (Liu, Insel, Reed, & Crist, 2012). Examining the process through which familism might exert its effects on outcome, Parveen et al. (2013) found that use of religious coping and positive reframing mediated the influence of familism on caregiver gains.

A study of South Asian elderly caregivers (Gupta & Pillai, 2002) found that the effect of role conflict on caregivers' perceived burden was significantly less in those with high levels of Asian filial piety, a construct related to familism. Such findings concur with other findings that suggest agreement with the caregiving expectancies of one's culture may mitigate negative perceptions of the caregiving role or perhaps the reporting of those perceptions (Coon et al., 2004; Gallagher-Thomson et al., 2003).

Conclusion

There is a clear need to examine caregiving within and not just between cultures. The assumption that there is little variation within one ethnic group or one culture limits the implications of the research for developing culturally sensitive services. Factors that differ within groups and that may affect caregiver outcomes include language, religion, caregiving, and support-seeking norms. Additionally, immigration and acculturation may influence caregiving and deserve research attention (Lord, Livingston, & Cooper, 2015). Generational differences in acculturation and in the traditional values and expectations regarding the care they are entitled to from their children exist within immigrant populations (Soskolne, Halevy-Levin, Cohen, & Friedman, 2006) and may explain some of the variation in the lived experience of caregiving across cultures and micro-cultures.

As described in Chapter 1, aspects of the illness context play a significant role in caregiver outcomes, yet the influence of illness perceptions of the caregiver has rarely been explored. The nature of the caregiving tasks is culturally relevant but rarely acknowledged. For example, even the large EUROFAMCARE review of informal care policy and practice uses the word "ethnicity" only five times in 150 pages (Mestheneos et al., 2005). The key mention is in an appendix, where three countries (Sweden, France, and Denmark) call for more research with ethnic groups and immigrants.

It is also worth considering that there is an overabundance in the caregiving literature of studies of dementia caregivers, a condition with quite different features than physical illnesses and with potentially different cultural explanations and responses. Further research is therefore needed before our understanding of the similarities and differences in the responses and outcomes of caregivers from different cultures, micro-cultures, ethnicities, and religions will be sufficient to inform culturally sensitive interventions and support services for both care recipients and caregivers. Moreover, researchers should not presuppose attitudinal or behavioral differences simply because a caregiver is of one particular culture. However, acknowledging that we function in a social world requires that at the very least, we examine these macro- and micro-cultural influences.

7
Personality and Caregiving

Revenson, Tracey A., Konstadina Griva, Aleksandra Luszczynska, Val Morrison, Efharis Panagopoulou, Noa Vilchinsky, and Mariët Hagedoorn. *Caregiving in the Illness Context*. Basingstoke: Palgrave Macmillan, 2016. DOI: 10.1057/9781137558985.0010.

Some caregivers acclimate better than others to the caregiving role, even when coping with similar threats to a loved one's health (Arenstein & Brown, 2014; Orgeta & Leung, 2015). Understanding why, through examining the underlying differences among individuals, may assist caregivers in adjusting to the difficult demands placed on them by serious chronic illnesses.

Personality traits, those consistent and unique individual biopsychosocial patterns of cognitions and behaviors (Friedman, 2011), are known to exert both direct and indirect effects on patients' psychological and physiological outcomes (Ferguson, 2013; Stanton, Revenson, & Tennen, 2007). Recently, growing scientific attention has been directed at testing the influence of personality on *caregiving* in the context of physical illness, including caregivers' motivation and ability to provide adequate care, the psychological and physiological outcomes of caregiving, and the reciprocal influence of caregivers' and care recipients' personalities (Lakey, 2013; Pietromonaco, Uchino, & Dunkel Schetter, 2013). Empirical findings testify to the power of personality theories in explaining how individuals will cope with various stressors during their lifetime, including caring for an ill loved one (Ferguson, 2013).

This chapter focuses on the five-factor model of personality (McCrae & Costa, 2003) and attachment orientations (e.g., Mikulincer & Shaver, 2007) as they have been the subject of most empirical studies in the caregiving context. In order to portray as full a picture as possible, positive aspects of personality and their relation to caregiving will be also reviewed. In this chapter we make the assumption that personality is considered to crystalize at young age and therefore to precede the caregiving situation. Evidence also exist for the opposite direction suggesting that personality may also be modified by the caregiving experience, although this is not covered in this chapter (Mikulincer, Ein-Dor, Solomon, & Shaver, 2011; Välimäki et al., 2014).

Personality constructs and their theoretical relation to caregiving

Personality can be defined as the "biopsychosocial patterns that make people uniquely themselves ..." (Friedman, 2011, p. 219). In other words, personality is the consistent and enduring set of traits or dispositions that are associated with particular patterns of cognitions, emotions, and behaviors (Orgeta & Leung, 2015). The inherent interplay among personality and caregiving may be explained via a number of well-established theoretical models. The basic premise of all these models is that caregivers are not born to be caregivers. The job does not come with a training manual; rather, in order to adjust to their newfound caregiving role, they instinctively fall back on pre-existing personality traits (McClendon & Smyth, 2013). Indeed, according to the stress-diathesis model of psychopathology (Monroe & Simons, 1991), negative psychological outcomes result from the joint effects of a diathesis – that is, a vulnerability or predisposition – and stressful experiences. Accordingly, individual differences in consequences for caregivers may be related to underlying personality dispositions, making them more or less vulnerable toward negative outcomes stemming from caregiving demands (Orgeta & Leung, 2015).

The five-factor model of personality

One of the most established conceptualizations of personality is the five-factor model (McCrae & Costa, 2003) which consists of neuroticism, conscientiousness, openness, extraversion, and agreeableness. The five-factor model suggests several pathways by which a specific personality orientation may affect an individual's adjustment to the caregiving role. For example, *neuroticism* contains the tendency to focus on the negative aspects of others and the world in general; greater neuroticism in caregivers may therefore be associated with the perception of the caregiving situation as difficult and demanding (Bookwala & Schulz, 1998). *Extraversion* might be associated with better mental health in the caregiving situation because this trait is characterized by an optimistic view of life and the ability to gather social support (Koerner, Kenyon, & Shirai, 2009). *Conscientiousness* – which includes planning ahead, organization, and meticulousness – might protect caregivers from feeling overwhelmed by the daily tasks and stressors associated with caregiving. Caregivers high on *agreeableness* – defined by characteristics such as being warm, caring, and helpful – might be more naturally suited to a caregiving role, and might therefore derive greater benefits from their caregiving efforts, than caregivers whose personalities are marked by emotional distance, lack of motivation to help, and/or indifference to others (Koerner et al., 2009). Finally, *openness* to experience which reflects the extent to which one is curious and imaginative may be related to better caregivers' outcomes due to the tendency to view the caregiving situation as a challenging new experience.

Attachment orientations

A personality theory that has accumulated much empirical evidence in the context of caregiving is the psychoanalytic theory of attachment, initially described by Bowlby (1973, 1982, 1988) and more recently widely disseminated by Mikulincer and Shaver (Mikulincer & Shaver, 2007, 2009; Shaver & Mikulincer, 2008). Attachment theory explains how repeated interactions between infant and caregiver result in an individual's lifelong ability to deal with – among other things – stress, illness, and caregiving (Maunder & Hunter, 2001, 2008). The main premise of attachment theory is that human beings are evolutionarily wired from birth to seek help, security, and solace from attachment figures who are expected to provide them with care and protection (Mikulincer & Shaver, 2007). Attachment theoreticians suggest that secure attachment is critical for responsive caregiving; insecure individuals, who fear abandonment and who did not receive the care they needed during their early years, bring their less-adaptable working models regarding how care is provided to the caregiving situation – a tendency which would likely color the kind of care they are able to provide others (Bowlby, 1982; Tsilika, Parpa, Zygogianni, Kouloulias, & Mystakidou, 2014).

According to attachment theory, a major stressor such as illness is especially likely to activate the attachment system; thus, the ability to cope with caring for an ill loved one will be determined, in part, by attachment orientation (J. A. Feeney & Ryan, 1994). Attachment is commonly conceptualized as two orientations: attachment anxiety ("hyper-activation of the attachment system") and avoidance ("deactivation of this system"). Individuals are considered securely attached if they score low on either dimension (Mikulincer & Shaver, 2007). Individuals with greater attachment security tend to provide care and support that is sensitive, cooperative, and warm. In contrast, more insecurely attached individuals are less likely to provide effective and sensitive support and care (Tsilika et al., 2014). For example, avoidant individuals' discomfort with closeness, excessive self-reliance, and lack of empathy seem to moderate the ability to provide sensitive and responsive caregiving (Mikulincer & Shaver, 2007; Van Assche et al., 2013). Caregivers who are high on anxious attachment tend to provide a kind of care that is focused more on self needs than partner needs, a result perhaps of the individual's anxiety about receiving less attention than the partner who is ill (Braun, Mikulincer, Rydall, Walsh, & Rodin,

2007; Karantzas, Evans, & Foddy, 2010; Mikulincer, Shaver, Gillath, & Nitzberg, 2005).

Stress-resistance resources

Several personality variables have been suggested to operate as stress-resistance resources (Ouellette & DiPlacido, 2001; Smith, Gallo, Shivpuri, & Brewer, 2012). Examples of these are mastery (Pearlin, Mullan, Semple, & Skaff, 1990; Skaff, Pearlin, & Mullan, 1996), dispositional optimism (Carver, Scheier, Miller, & Fulford, 2009), sense of coherence (Antonovsky, 1993), and hardiness (Kobasa, Maddi, & Kahn, 1982).

According to the stress and coping framework (Lazarus & Folkman, 1984) described in Chapter 2, cognitive appraisal is the key to understanding the effects of stressors on an individual's well-being. Personality shapes these cognitive appraisals of stress. Depending on personality, some caregivers may perceive that they are under more stress than others, even in relatively equivalent caregiving situations. For example, stronger beliefs about personal control and mastery are associated with a tendency to interpret the environment as less stressful (Folkman, 1984; Lazarus & Folkman, 1984). Thus, caregivers characterized by low levels of mastery may assess the caregiving situation as more difficult and burdensome than caregivers high on mastery and personal control (Bookwala & Schulz, 1998).

According to Carver and Scheier's self-regulation theory (Carver & Scheier, 1998), dispositional optimism plays an important role in an individual's ability to cope with life's ups and downs. More optimistic people are more likely to keep goals in mind and work persistently toward achieving those goals, the result of which is the achievement of more positive outcomes over time (Hooker, Monahan, Bowman, Frazier, & Shifren, 1998). Thus, it is reasonable to expect that more optimistic individuals would adjust better to the caregiving situation.

Both hardiness and sense of coherence are personality constructs based on health – enhancing, or what Antonovsky (1993) termed "salutogenic effects", on coping with stressful life contexts (Clark & Hartman, 1996). Hardiness is defined as the predisposition to feel committed to one's life, view change as challenge, and to have a sense of control over one's life (Kobasa et al., 1982). Sense of coherence (SOC) stands for the tendency to perceive the world as comprehensive, manageable, and meaningful (Antonovsky, 1993). Thus, both hardiness and SOC may be conceptualized as internal resources.

The relation between personality and caregiving outcomes

Personality and the motivation and ability to provide care

Different personality traits have been associated with both the inclination to provide care at all, as well as with being able to provide it in an adequate way. The ability to provide effective care starts with an accurate appraisal of the partner's suffering – an appraisal which, as portrayed in the previous section, may be determined to a great extent by one's personality characteristics. Indeed, Bookwala and Schulz (1998) found that coronary heart patient caregivers who had higher neuroticism scores perceived more difficulties in the execution of their caregiving tasks than caregivers lower on neuroticism.

Attachment avoidance has been related to less caregiving overall, less instrumental care (Carnelley, Pietromonaco, & Jaffe, 1996), and difficulty in providing care (Kunce & Shaver, 1994). Attachment security was found, among caregivers of cancer patients, to be positively related to autonomous motives for caregiving (i.e., those motives which derive from the self rather than from social pressures). Attachment anxiety, however, was related to "introjected" motives (i.e., behaving in a certain way in order to avoid shame or guilt (Kim, Carver, Deci, & Kasser, 2008).

Regarding the quality of care, neuroticism was related to less-adaptive caregiving strategies (including impatience, anger, and withdrawing) among caregivers of individuals with dementia (De Vugt et al., 2004). In a cross-sectional survey of family caregivers of individuals with dementia (McClendon & Smyth, 2013), higher levels of agreeableness, conscientiousness, openness and – contrary to predictions – neuroticism, were associated with high quality care (i.e., care that was respectful, supportive, personalized, and marked by less withdrawal). Greater levels of extraversion, however, were associated with greater controlling and withdrawal behaviors by the caregiver. The authors suggested that extraversion may have increased withdrawal behaviors because it consists of a tendency toward hypervigilance or assertiveness (McClendon & Smyth, 2013).

Evidence from laboratory studies indicates that people high on the attachment avoidance orientation are likely to be less sensitive and responsive to their partner's needs (B. C. Feeney & Collins, 2001). Those high on the attachment anxiety orientation tend to engage in overinvolved and controlling forms of caregiving (B. C. Feeney & Collins, 2001). Studies performed in natural settings with caregivers have shown similar patterns. For example, attachment anxiety has been associated with the provision of more problematic care for cognitively and physically impaired care recipients (Morse, Shaffer, Williamson, Dooley, & Schulz, 2012).

Personality and adjustment to the caregiver role

In this section we focus on the spectrum of caregivers' own adjustment to their new role as care providers, paying particular attention to caregivers' burden and mental and physical health.

Mental health outcomes. A substantial body of literature has found that neuroticism is significantly related to poorer mental health (i.e., depression and anxiety) among caregivers of patients with a variety of illlnesses: dementia, Alzheimer's disease, and Parkinson's disease (Gallant & Connell, 2003; Hooker et al., 1998; Hooker, Monahan, Shifren, & Hutchinson, 1992; Orgeta & Leung, 2015; Vedhara, Shanks, Wilcock, & Lightman, 2001); older adults with multiple functional problems (Löckenhoff, Duberstein, Friedman, & Costa, 2011); patients with coronary heart disease (Bookwala & Schulz, 1998; Patrick & Hayden, 1999; Ruiz, Matthews, Scheier, & Schulz, 2006); and cancer patients (Kim, Duberstein, Sörensen, & Larson, 2005; Nijboer, Tempelaar, Triemstra, van den Bos, & Sanderman, 2001). Far fewer scientific findings have been detected with regard to the other four factors of the five-factor model. In some studies extraverted caregivers exhibited fewer negative emotions, less depression, and better mental health than introverted caregivers (Jylha & Isometsa, 2006; Steel, Schmidt, & Shultz, 2008). However, this association has not been found in other studies (Löckenhoff et al., 2011). A word of caution is required here since many measures of neuroticism are similar to measures of depressive symptoms and mental health problems, which may create the high correlations and lack of discriminant validity (Smith, Williams, & Segerstrom, 2015).

Overall, both attachment anxiety and avoidance have been associated with poorer mental health, including measures of negative affectivity, and lower well-being (Nelis, Clare, & Whitaker, 2012; Porter et al., 2012; Tsilika et al., 2014). This association was detected among caregivers of patients coping with a broad range of illnesses, including dementia (Perren, Schmid, Herrmann, & Wettstein, 2007), cancer (Braun et al., 2007; Kim, Kashy, & Evans, 2007), and cognitive or physical impairments (Morse et al., 2012).

Finally, a handful of studies have detected that low levels of mastery, self-efficacy, self-esteem, perceived control and optimism have been associated with poorer mental health among caregivers (Bastawrous, Gignac, Kapral, & Cameron, 2014; Bookwala & Schulz, 1998; Dracup et al., 2004; Halm & Bakas, 2007; Hooker et al., 1992; Keefe et al., 2003; Kim et al., 2005; Nijboer et al., 2001; O'Dwyer, Moyle, Zimmer-Gembeck, & De Leo, 2013; Schmall, 1995).

Caregiver burden. Caregiver burden is defined as the extent to which caregivers perceive their emotional or physical health, social life, or financial status to be affected by their caring for an ill relative (Zarit, Todd, & Zarit, 1986). Numerous studies support the idea that caregivers' personality traits are associated with their level of (perceived) caregiving burden across illness domains. Overall, neuroticism has been related to greater caregiver burden, whereas extraversion and agreeableness have been associated with lower caregiver burden (Gonzalez-Abraldes, Millan-Calenti, Lorenzo-Lopez, & Maseda, 2013; Melo, Maroco, & De Mendonça, 2011; Shurgot & Knight, 2005). Recently low levels of sense of coherence were found to be associated with higher levels of burden among caregivers of stroke patients (Jaracz et al., 2015).

Personality traits have also been shown to moderate the association between burden and mental health. In a study of couples coping with a husband's heart attack, Vilchinsky and colleagues (2015) detected that female caregivers' burden was associated with less psychological distress among more secure caregivers, that is, those caregivers low on attachment anxiety. In studies of cancer caregivers, the negative impact of burden on mental health was weaker for caregivers high on the personality dispositions of self-efficacy, resilience, and optimism (Cassidy, Mclaughlin, & Giles, 2015; Kim et al., 2005).

Finding benefits in the caregiving experience. Burden and poor mental health are not the only possible outcome of caregiving; on the other end of the spectrum are the benefits that can be gained from the caregiving situation (see Chapter 2). Both agreeableness and extraversion have been significantly associated with the experience of caregiving benefits (Koerner et al., 2009); in contrast, neuroticism and conscientiousness were either not associated at all (Koerner et al., 2009) or, in the case of neuroticism, even negatively associated with the perception of the caregiving experience as positive (Hollis-Sawyer, 2001).

Attachment security has been related to benefit-finding among caregivers of cancer patients (Kim et al., 2005). Somewhat surprisingly, avoidance attachment was associated with finding meaning in the caregiving situation, but only for male caregivers (Hasson-Ohayon et al., 2013).

Physical health outcomes. Relatively few studies have focused on the contribution of caregivers' personality predispositions to the toll on caregivers' physical health. In the few studies that exist, the results show that some personality traits play a crucial role in the emergence of negative physical outcomes and morbidity among caregivers. For example, neuroticism was directly associated with poorer subjectively reported and objective physical health among Alzheimer's caregivers (Hooker et al., 1998, 1992; Monahan & Hooker, 1995). These associations may be attributed to the finding that neuroticism has been associated with fewer health-promoting behaviors among caregivers (Gallant & Connell, 2003). By contrast, conscientiousness was associated with fewer chronic health conditions (Hooker et al., 1992). Neither openness nor agreeableness were found to be associated with subjective physical health among caregivers (Hooker et al., 1992).

Low self-efficacy was associated with strong physiological reactions to the demands of caregiving among those caring for older people (Schmall, 1995). The same pattern was observed with regard to low mastery and physical fatigue among caregivers of older people with Alzheimer's disease (Roepke et al., 2009). Depression mediated the association between self-efficacy and cumulative health risk among caregivers of older people with dementia (Rabinowitz, Saenz, Thompson, & Gallagher-Thompson, 2011). Mausbach and colleagues (2011) found that when dementia caregivers' self-efficacy was low, caregiving overload was significantly related to IL-6, a known risk marker for health morbidity, particularly cardiovascular disease.

Personality, social support, and accepting care

It is well established that any support transaction, including the caregiver-care recipient dyad, must be regarded as a social interaction involving both caregiver and care-recipient (Chapter 1; Nelis et al., 2012; Revenson & DeLongis, 2011). Personality may facilitate or hinder not only the ability to provide care but also the ability to accept and benefit from it (Reinhardt, Boerner, & Horowitz, 2006). The personality of the care *receiver* therefore also plays a major role in the caregiving process.

Studies show that patients' personalities contribute both to their ability to seek and accept support and care (Cohen et al., 2005; Monin, Schulz, & Kershaw, 2013) and to benefit from it, in terms of lower levels of distress (Braun et al., 2007; Vilchinsky et al., 2010). The care recipient's personality may even have an effect on the caregiver's ability and motivation to provide care (Tsilika et al., 2014) and on caregiver outcomes such as burden (Magai & Cohen, 1998; Ruiz et al., 2006).

Conclusion

Personality traits have been consistently associated with caregiving-related variables such as the ability to adequately provide care, as well as caregivers' own psychological and physiological outcomes. Overall, personality traits that are considered maladaptive, such as neuroticism and having an insecure attachment orientation, are associated with negative caregiving outcomes and difficulties in providing care. Positive traits, such as secure attachment, agreeableness, optimism, mastery, self-esteem, and self-efficacy are mostly associated with better outcomes.

There does seem to be one exception to this rule. It seems that individuals high on neuroticism or anxious attachment may feel more obligated to enter into the caregiving role. Less emotionally stable individuals are more likely to assume caregiving responsibilities, most likely because of their tendency to be more worrisome and vigilant to stress communications coming from their partners (Rohr, Wagner, & Lang, 2013). According to attachment theoreticians, anxiously attached individuals tend to provide support and care that is compulsive in nature, rather than sensitive to a partner's needs, due to their urgent need to ease their own overwhelming distress (Mikulincer & Shaver, 2007). Thus, despite their being more engaged in caregiving acts, these individuals usually utilize less-adaptable coping strategies (Jin, Van Yperen, Sanderman, & Hagedoorn, 2010; Rohr et al., 2013).

These findings and others highlight the need for a better integration of personality with caregiving in the illness context. Understanding caregivers' personality may lead to the design of more effective interventions for caregivers (Monin et al., 2013). It is important to note that we are not proposing interventions that change personality; such a goal is neither feasible nor useful and may even lead to resentment among caregivers who seek professional help. What we do suggest is that interventions designed to help caregivers cope and ameliorate their distress be specifically adapted to caregivers' unique personality characteristics. For example, caregivers high on the avoidance attachment continuum may benefit more from psycho-education than from support groups, due to their rigid self-reliance. On the other hand, support groups may be just the right venue for the highly anxiously attached caregiver, who longs for attention and containment.

This chapter focused mainly on a small set of personality dispositions, ignoring others that may be important but have not received research attention. More importantly, we focused solely on the caregiver's personality. As the care recipient's personality also plays a major role in the caregiving inter-personal process, it is crucial to view the relationship between personality and care processes from the interactive perspectives of both those providing the care as well as those receiving it. As constructing the meaning of caregiving is dependent on one's personality predispositions, personality must be included in models of the caregiving process.

8
Interventions to Support Caregivers

Revenson, Tracey A., Konstadina Griva, Aleksandra Luszczynska, Val Morrison, Efharis Panagopoulou, Noa Vilchinsky, and Mariët Hagedoorn. *Caregiving in the Illness Context*. Basingstoke: Palgrave Macmillan, 2016.
DOI: 10.1057/9781137558985.0011.

Suboptimal support of caregivers may have several deleterious consequences. These include turning to formal care needed to address the patient's medical and personal care needs and possible services to maintain the mental and physical health of caregivers, both involve additional financial burden (Mittleman, 2005). As patients' needs grow and their dependence on caregivers increases, the caregivers' ability to maintain a high level of care may be affected. Therefore, interventions addressing the psychosocial needs of caregivers may improve patient as well as caregiver outcomes, and decrease economic costs related to the use of health services (Mittleman, 2005).

A number of theory- and evidence-based interventions have been developed to enhance caregivers' health and well-being, minimize the negative effects of caregiving on caregivers, and optimize outcomes for patients. Attempts to categorize interventions distinguish practical support intervention (e.g., respite interventions) from information and education interventions (targeting knowledge and skills of caregivers), and from psychological or psychosocial support interventions (targeting caregivers' health directly (Kayser & Scott, 2008; Legg et al., 2011; Tong, Sainsbury, & Craig, 2008).

This chapter provides an overview of these three categories of interventions. To illustrate the trends in recent research we focus on reporting findings obtained in systematic reviews and meta-analyses that provide an overarching synthesis of high-quality studies. We discuss the content of the interventions, their effectiveness, satisfaction, feasibility, reach, and cultural issues.

Practical support – respite services

Respite services aim at improvement of the caregivers' well-being through providing a temporary break in their care activities. Respite care takes many forms, including adult day care, institutional respite, or a host family respite. In each form of respite the care recipient is taken care of by someone else while the caregiver gets a bit of restoration (Mason et al., 2007). In the United States, publicly funded respite services may be available for caregivers of older persons with chronic illness (Mason et al., 2007).

A review of randomized controlled trials (RCTs) of day care programs for older people with chronic health issues indicated that only half of the 22 reviewed trials showed a significant positive effect on caregiver outcomes (Mason et al., 2007). The evidence from non-RCT studies (e.g., studies without a control group or random assignment) is stronger, with at least one caregiver outcome improved in each study, including burnout, depression, freedom, relaxation, or satisfaction. Similar mixed findings were observed in studies examining other types of respite services (Mason et al., 2007). Overall, a meta-analysis indicated that different types of respite care did not reduce caregiver burden although a small, significant reduction of depressive symptoms was found (Mason et al., 2007). Importantly, when satisfaction with respite services was evaluated, caregivers appeared to be more satisfied with respite care than with standard care (e.g., an education and counseling session; Mason et al., 2007).

A review of studies on caregivers of community-dwelling elders showed that respite services may be effective in reducing depression, stress, and role strain, but they did not improve caregivers' quality of life (QOL; Lopez-Hartmann, Wens, Verhoeven, & Remmen, 2012). These results may stem from the fact that participation in respite care does not mean that the caregivers are withdrawing or reducing their regular caring activities. Even after placing their relative in assisted care, more than a half of caregivers perform tasks similar to those carried out when the patient was living at home (Schulz et al., 2014).

Information and educational interventions

When faced with either acute care demands (e.g., post-stroke, acute myocardial infarction) or increased care demands (e.g., a deterioration of the patient's condition) caregivers may struggle to adequately perform caregiving duties. The resulting strain can have deleterious effects for the caregiver not only directly but also indirectly through the patient's increased health problems, increased anxiety, and decreased QOL (Gemmill & Cooke, 2011).

One of the major aims of educational interventions is the improvement of skills and knowledge for managing the illness, as well as the improvement of caregivers' understanding of patients' functioning (Gemmill & Cooke, 2011). These interventions may improve caregivers' well-being by increasing their sense of control, mastery and self-efficacy, and by reducing confusion and uncertainty. In this way they increase the caregiver's preparedness to deal with new medical or care issues as they arise

(Gemmill & Cooke, 2011). Skills and knowledge interventions usually take place when the patient is still hospitalized (e.g., after hip fracture or stroke; Forster et al., 2015) or following hospitalization (Martín-Martín et al., 2014). Alternately, they may be delivered to caregivers who have long-term experience in caring for patients with chronic illness who need a refresher or when new demands arise (Tong et al., 2008).

Caregiving for a person with a chronic illness, and thus specific needs, can be considered a *unique experience* (Aoun et al., 2012). Each illness – its consequences, timeline, and progression (Leventhal et al., 2012) – is often unique and the course of intervention unpredictable. These facts may be either unknown to caregivers, difficult to understand, or hard to predict as many illnesses have a variable course. Therefore, the educational interventions are most effective when they highlight the skills and knowledge tailored to the specific illness and the key needs of specific patients and caregivers (Aoun et al., 2012). Interventions may teach caregiver skills to identify problem areas and make adaptations in the patients' environment, for example to prevent falls or to increase of patients' mobility (Martín-Martín et al., 2014).

For example, caregivers of stroke patients learn about the consequences of stroke and stroke-related problems, dietary needs and feeding techniques, communication techniques if the care recipient has dysphasia, and personal care tasks such as washing, dressing, limb positioning, and management of pressure areas (Forster et al., 2015). For couples facing prostate cancer post-surgery, caregivers may need to learn how to clean the catheter, look for signs of infection, and maintain fluid intake (Diefenbach et al., 2015). In the case of caregivers who provide assistance to patients with motor neuron diseases, central aspects of the intervention include the need for almost continual care; understanding of cognitive and neurobehavioral decline; assisted ventilation; end-of-life caregiving and requests for hastened death; and bereavement (Aoun et al., 2012).

Psychosocial support interventions to reduce stress and burden

The interventions in this category are based on increasing caregivers' emotion management and problem-solving skills, combining multiple intervention strategies in a package. A systematic review of the interventions aiming at an improvement of QOL among caregivers of cancer patients (Waldron, Janke, Bechtel, Ramirez, & Cohen, 2013) showed that 83% of the interventions offered education on patient and caregiver outcomes, 66% addressed relationship problems, 66% addressed communication between caregivers and patients, 33% interventions included coping skills training, 33% addressed skills to improve sleep habits, and 17% addressed problem-solving.

Problem-solving is one of the most frequently used interventions (see Gemmill & Cooke, 2011, for an example with transplant patients). Interventions that address problem-solving may rely on complex frameworks. The COPE framework, for example, includes four components:

- Creativity: viewing a stressful problem from various perspectives to find alternative coping strategies and solutions.
- Optimism: the ability to have a positive attitude.
- Planning: setting reasonably attainable goals.
- Expert information: able to make a decision about when to access professional help.

In many interventions, problem-solving is combined with other techniques, for example aiming at an improvement of caregivers' communication skills and coping with burden (Northouse, Williams, Given, & McCorkle, 2012). In another study, caregivers of allogeneic hematopoietic stem cell transplant patients who attended a multi-session intervention aimed at stress management, breathing, and enhancing social support receipt showed lower caregiver stress, depression, and anxiety three months post-transplant than those who received usual care (Laudenslager et al., 2015). This time point was meaningful because it is the point post-transplant when the caregiver is assuming a 24/7 burden.

Among telehealth-based interventions for caregivers, 37% included educational components, 37% taught decision-making strategies, 35% used the elements of problem-solving training and cognitive-behavioral treatment elements, and 23% focused on social support provision and receipt (Chi & Demiris, 2015). Web-based interventions for caregivers of cancer patients often contain multiple components as well, including information (about illness and available resources), communication skills, self-regulation, optimism, coping effectiveness, uncertainty reduction, and symptom management (Kaltenbaugh et al., 2015). The interventions targeting caregivers of patients at the end-of-life often focus on caregivers' coping skills, including problem-solving (Goy, 2012).

Psychosocial interventions may also address relationship-related sources of stress, such as deficits or mutuality in the relationships between caregiver and the patient (Gemmill & Cooke, 2011). Among various well-being interventions for caregivers of cancer patients, approximately 17% focused primarily on strengthening patient-caregiver relationship, managing conflicts in the relationship, and dealing with loss (Northouse et al., 2012).

Dyadic interventions for patients with chronic illnesses involve both the patient and caregiver together. They often address communication skills of both partners as well as joint problem-solving skills (Kayser & Scott, 2008; Northouse et al., 2012), which have been shown in other studies to enhance adaptation (e.g., Badr, Carmack, Kashy, Cristofanilli, & Revenson, 2010). Dyadic interventions have been studied most frequently among cancer patients (see reviews by Badr & Krebs, 2013; Brandão, Schulz, & Matos, 2014; Martire, Schulz, Helgeson, Small, & Saghafi, 2010). Dyadic interventions delivered in the context of cancer usually consist of multiple components and include education of the patients and their partners regarding illness management, enhancement of communication or support, relationship functioning, and elements of cognitive-behavioral training. For example, interventions for patients with cancer and their partners may use techniques derived from interpersonal counseling, behavioral marital therapy, emotion-focused therapy, cognitive-behavioral therapy, and education (Badr & Krebs, 2013). Those techniques are used to strengthen individual, communal, or dyadic coping, joint problem-solving, coordinating everyday demands, the use of relationship-related resources, and approaching cancer together as a team. One meta-analysis found that dyadic interventions had significantly larger positive effects on well-being when the target group included cancer patients and their caregivers, compared to interventions for caregivers and patients with cardiovascular diseases (Hartmann, Baezner, Wild, Eisler, & Herzog, 2010).

Self-care interventions that promote caregivers' physical health

Balancing the care responsibilities and patients' needs with caregivers' own needs is a challenging task (Gemmill & Cooke, 2011), creating a need for self-care interventions that keep the caregiver healthy while under much stress. The number of studies of self-care interventions is limited, but all of them showed a significant reduction of stress or an improvement in QOL (Gemmill & Cooke, 2011). For example, in the context of hematopoietic cell transplant, self-care interventions for caregivers include yoga, relaxation techniques, massage, and behavioral techniques aiming at improving sleep (Gemmill & Cooke, 2011). Despite their importance, caregivers' diet and exercise are addressed relatively rarely. For example, only 1 in 33 dyadic interventions conducted in the context of cancer care targeted a change in caregivers' diet and body weight (Martire et al., 2010). In case of caregivers of older adults with chronic health problems, respite intervention has been combined with an intervention targeting caregivers' well-being (Schulz et al., 2014). In addition to addressing caregivers' mental health and providing information about how care will change across the illness trajectory, self-care interventions address issues of end-of-life care and end-of-life planning (Schulz et al., 2014). Interventions for caregivers of newly admitted hospice patients address care over the final months, and even the final days, of life (Lindstrom & Mazurek-Melnyk, 2013), including information about how to handle symptoms and pain as well as what to expect in terms of one's own anxiety, depression, and preparedness for end-of-life.

Effectiveness of interventions

One of the first reviews to investigate the effectiveness of interventions for caregivers suggested that the evidence is mixed and our understanding of the effects of the interventions on health and well-being outcomes is limited (Harding & Higginson, 2003). Reviews conducted a decade later still show that the effects are mixed and often small but offer more promise (e.g., Badr & Krebs, 2013)

There are several systematic reviews and meta-analyses examining the effects of the interventions on caregiver outcomes (Badr & Krebs, 2013; Brandão et al., 2014; Martire et al., 2010). The findings differ as a result of study design; some reviews include only RCTs whereas other reviews include quasi-experimental and observational studies. The findings also differ depending on the type(s) of illness included, the types of interventions, their delivery method, and the outcomes assessed. We will summarize the findings by caregiver outcome, as we did in Chapter 2.

Quality of life

A review of high-grade RCTs that studied the effectiveness of interventions targeting stroke patients and their caregivers showed that only one in eight interventions resulted in a significant increase in QOL (Legg et al., 2011). The distinctive characteristic of the successful interventions referred to care skills training. Another systematic review evaluating interventions for caregivers of stroke survivors concluded that education and psychosocial programs were effective in improving caregivers' QOL (Corry, While, Neenan, & Smith, 2015). A review of interventions for caregivers of cancer patients showed that caregivers' QOL improved significantly in 33% of the studies and the effects were observed at follow-ups three to four months later (Waldron et al., 2013). A review of dyadic interventions for couples coping with cancer came to a similar conclusion, with a weighted effect size of .25 (Badr & Krebs, 2013). Another review of dyadic interventions for patients with cancer and their partners showed that a majority of interventions had a positive effect on at least one area of partner's QOL (Brandão et al., 2014). In contrast, most studies of interventions for caregivers of patients at the end-of-life stage showed no significant change in caregiver QOL (Goy, 2012). Among telehealth interventions, QOL improvements were shown in 12% of 65 studies (Chi & Demiris, 2015).

Depression, anxiety, stress, and caregiver burden

Most reviews focus on a specific illness condition. A review of high-grade trials investigating effectiveness of interventions targeting caregivers and stroke patients showed no effects of interventions on anxiety, and a small percentage (about 13%) showed a reduction in caregivers' stress or strain (Legg et al., 2011). Another review of stroke caregivers found mixed results with depression and caregiver burden (Corry et al., 2015) and yet another review of RCTs for family interventions for caregivers and stroke patients showed no effects on caregiver burden or depression (Cheng, Chair, & Chau, 2014).

A review of interventions for caregivers of patients with chronic kidney diseases yielded mixed results regarding burden and stress (Tong et al., 2008). The majority of interventions targeting caregivers of patients at the end-of-life were also effective in reducing caregivers' distress (Goy, 2012). A review of dyadic interventions for caregivers and patients with a chronic illness showed that 35% of interventions were effective in reducing stress or anxiety (Martire et al., 2010).

An analysis of telehealth interventions showed that most frequently investigated outcomes referred to anxiety, depression, stress, burden, or irritability (Chi & Demiris, 2015). In particular, 44% of 65 reviewed studies indicated a significant reduction in caregivers' anxiety, depression, stress, burden, or irritability (Chi & Demiris, 2015). Among web-based multicomponent interventions for caregivers of cancer patients (Kaltenbaugh et al., 2015), 60% resulted in a significant reduction of negative affect, but the number of studies reviewed was very small, limiting conclusions.

Social and family functioning

Interventions for caregivers of stroke survivors showed mixed findings regarding social or family functioning (Corry et al., 2015). The review focusing on family interventions for caregivers and stroke patients showed small positive effects on family functioning (Cheng et al., 2014). The review of dyadic interventions for caregivers and patients with a chronic illness showed that 35% of these interventions resulted in significant and consistent changes in perceptions of marital quality and coping as a couple (Martire et al., 2010). Again, few of the telehealth interventions (14%) showed significant positive effects, and these effects were primarily on perceptions of social support, improved social functioning, and meeting needs for social support or social interaction (Chi & Demiris, 2015).

Competence and mastery

A review of education interventions for caregivers of stroke survivors showed that programs were effective in improving caregivers' competence evaluations (Corry et al., 2015). Yet, a review of RCTs focusing on family interventions for caregivers of stroke patients indicated no significant effects on self-evaluations of competency or adequacy of own caregiver performance (Cheng et al., 2014). A review of studies evaluating interventions for caregivers of patients with brain cancer (high-grade gliomas) indicated that psychoeducational programs may increase feelings of mastery among caregivers (Piil, Juhler, Jakobsen, & Jarden, 2014), but these conclusions were based on findings from one trial only. Interventions focusing on caregivers' knowledge were found to significantly influence participants' understanding and knowledge about illness and care for patients with chronic kidney diseases (Tong et al., 2008). The review of dyadic interventions (delivered in the context of a chronic illness) showed that only 35% of all interventions yielded consistent improvements in self-efficacy and mastery (Martire et al., 2010). The majority of interventions targeting caregivers of patients at the end-of-life resulted in negligible changes in perceptions of ability to deal with caregiver role demands (Goy, 2012). Approximately 20% of telehealth interventions result in an improvement of caregiver knowledge, skills, or competence in managing patient's symptoms (Chi & Demiris, 2015).

Physical health

The effects of interventions on caregivers' physical health and physical functioning have been investigated much less and the evidence is decidedly mixed. A meta-analysis addressing the physical health of family caregivers of cancer patients showed a significant improvement of physical functioning among intervention participants compared to the standard care (Northouse et al., 2012). However, across dyadic interventions for caregivers and patients with a chronic illness, only 12% (four trials) considered the physical health of caregivers (Martire et al., 2010) and all but one showed a positive effect on partner's health (better self-reported health, greater weight loss). A review focusing on family interventions for caregivers and stroke patients showed no significant effects on somatic complaints (Cheng et al., 2014).

Limitations of the research

The first issue in evaluating the effectiveness of the interventions refers to the multiplicity of outcomes. Interventions for caregivers of patients with physical disability showed that the evaluation often included multiple primary and secondary outcomes (Lawanag, Horey, Blackford, Sunsern, & Riewpaiboon, 2013). As a result, all interventions had a positive effect on at least one of the outcomes (Lawanag et al., 2013; Lopez-Hartmann et al., 2012). For example, among telehealth technology based interventions, 95% resulted in an improvement of at least one outcome and only 5% did not find improvement on any outcome (Chi & Demiris, 2015). Thus, having multiple interrelated outcomes might create spurious findings.

Another issue is the consistency of the findings, that is, did the intervention have a positive influence across all the outcomes in one study (Lopez-Hartmann et al., 2012)? For example, compared to usual care, only one in three of dyadic interventions evaluated by Martire et al. (2010) resulted in consistent effects on caregivers' outcomes.

The significant effects of interventions are more likely to be found when interventions are compared with waiting list controls rather than active "usual care" control group, that was receiving at least minimal education and informational support (Corry et al., 2015; Lawang, Horey, Blackforf, Sunsern, & Riewpaiboon, 2013). The high-evidence grade studies (e.g., RCTs) resulted in a significant improvement in only some caregiver outcomes or in no effects at all compared to observational studies (Harding, List, Epiphaniou, & Jones, 2011). Moreover, in those RCT trials that did show effects, the effect sizes were small (Badr & Krebs, 2013; Lopez-Hartmann et al., 2012; Schulz et al., 2014) and improvement was more likely to occur if the outcomes were measured a short time after the intervention was completed (Harding et al., 2011; Schulz et al., 2014). Stated another way, most of the significant effects were for short term; they were not long-term effects.

Forming conclusions about intervention efficacy is very difficult, as a result of the diversity of interventions in terms of study designs, target populations, and different content or format of interventions. The strongest conclusions may be drawn from Northouse et al.'s (2012) review of reviews discussing the effects of interventions for caregivers of patients with various chronic illnesses. Overall, caregivers who received an intervention, compared to controls, reported significantly less burden, less depression, and less distress; they also reported more knowledge, better coping, greater mental well-being, and better quality of life. The effect sizes varied from small to medium and often occurred shortly after the completion of the intervention program, for example, at three months follow-up. Moreover, preliminary evidence indicated that intervention effectiveness may be moderated by type: Two meta-analyses found that interventions designed to improve caregivers' knowledge had larger effects on patient or caregiver outcomes than those designed to decrease caregivers' depression (Northouse, Katapodi, Song, Zhang, & Mood, 2010; Sörensen, Pinquart, & Duberstein, 2002).

Delivery of interventions

Interventions may be delivered to both patient and caregiver or to a caregiver alone. Rates of dyadic interventions range from 37% for telehealth interventions (Chi & Demiris, 2015) to 50–60% for in-person interventions (Waldron et al., 2013; Northouse et al., 2012).

The majority of programs have components that are delivered face-to-face or combine in-person and telephone-based delivery (Legg et al., 2011); fewer interventions use a group format. Overall, the majority of interventions were delivered by health care professionals (e.g., nurses, psychologists). Among interventions for caregivers of cancer patients, the most frequently applied formats include groups or individual interventions, most often delivered by nurses (Harding et al., 2011; Lawanag et al., 2013; Waldron et al., 2013).

The dose of the interventions varies, with some programs including 2 meetings and lasting less than 2 hours (Northouse et al., 2012) to 16 sessions lasting 18 hours (Northouse et al., 2012). Another review found that dyadic interventions took between 3 and 20 sessions (Martire et al., 2010).

Face-to-face interventions using group or individual meeting formats are time-consuming, may be expensive, and require either taking time off work or care-related responsibilities (Kaltenbaugh et al., 2015). Therefore, programs involving face-to-face meetings may reach only a fraction of caregivers. Alternative forms of delivery, in particular web-based or other telehealth interventions (e.g., videoconferencing, telephone, web) offer a way to improve access (Chi & Demiris, 2015).

Satisfaction, feasibility, and reach

Feasibility, acceptability, and satisfaction with the intervention are seldom evaluated (Legg et al., 2011). In one systematic review, caregivers of stroke patients reported greater satisfaction with their understanding of the causes of stroke, but there were negligible differences in satisfaction with one's own skills and knowledge for preventing another stroke (Legg et al., 2011). Another review of family interventions for stroke survivors found that caregivers who participated in psychoeducational interventions (individual or group format) reported higher satisfaction than those in the control groups (Cheng et al., 2014); however, satisfaction was assessed in only 17% of the studies. Among 65 telehealth interventions evaluated by Chi and Demiris (2015), 38% of the studies showed an improvement in the caregiver's confidence and satisfaction with their participation. Furthermore, a lack of satisfaction was accompanied by a lack of improvement – in health or well-being. In case of web-based multicomponent interventions for caregivers of cancer patients, the feasibility of interventions is seldom (only 17% of studies; Kaltenbaugh et al., 2015).

There are several small-scale observational studies that evaluate caregivers' satisfaction with an intervention. These studies indicate that participants may be satisfied with helpfulness of the intervention team, information received, resources available, and opportunities to meet other caregivers, even if there are no improvements shown. For example, an intervention study for caregivers of leukemia patients showed high caregiver satisfaction with the intervention (Pailler et al., 2015); however, because the study did not have a usual care group, it is not known whether the intervention had any effects. Caregivers of hospice patients who took part in an intervention addressing end-of-life issues perceived the intervention as feasible and acceptable (Lindstrom & Mazurek-Melnyk, 2013).

Securing broad reach and low attrition is an important good practice characteristic of interventions (Horodyska et al., 2015). A review of interventions for caregivers of patients in palliative care showed that the programs have problems with recruitment and attendance (Harding & Higginson, 2003). High attrition rates among caregivers of patients with more serious disease indicated that the programs might be too burdensome for the participants (Piil et al., 2014). Finally, reaching caregivers from rural regions may be difficult if regular face-to-face meetings are required, but easier and more feasible with telehealth interventions. However, only 23% of the interventions using Internet or phone-based technologies target rural caregivers (Chi & Demiris, 2015).

Cultural issues in interventions

To date, the role of how cultural factors influence caregiver or dyadic interventions has not been systematically investigated, yet we need that evidence to design culturally anchored interventions. Most of the research has been conducted in North America, Europe, Asia, and Australia (Harding et al., 2011). This is one area where US-based research is not dominating the field; for example, only 22% of interventions for caregivers providing assistance to patients with motor neuron diseases were conducted in the United States (Aoun et al., 2012). There are a few reviews of interventions in particular countries or cultures (e.g., Thai family caregivers, Lawanag et al., 2013, and caregivers of people with chronic kidney disease in Spain or India, Tong et al., 2008). Telehealth interventions seem to be more popular in the United States than in other countries (Chi & Demiris, 2015) but this may soon change.

Future directions for research, policy, and practice

Current interventions for caregivers are lacking in several ways. First, there is need for more precision in identifying the specific techniques for problem-solving. Interventions using "problem-solving techniques" may in fact combine different techniques, such as enhancing optimism and self-efficacy or teaching the caregiver to create action plans for coping. The reports of the interventions often lack details allowing for identifying the specific components of the interventions and the ways these components were delivered. This information is crucial for understanding the ways the interventions influence caregivers' well-being (see Abraham, Johnson, de Bruin, & Luszczynska, 2014).

Second, the theoretical background underlying many interventions is often absent or unstated. Many interventions refer to a "cognitive-behavioral approach" as the theoretical framework (Waldron et al., 2013), but do not specify which aspects in the cognitive-behavioral approach are implemented. Finally, research almost never investigates the underlying mechanisms that may explain *why* the intervention should influence the desired outcomes or determine which of the intervention's components are responsible for the change in the outcomes. Therefore, even if a caregiver intervention is shown to be effective in a well-designed study, we do not know why.

This brings us to future work. One of the main issues requiring investigation refers to the medical of caregivers (Aoun et al., 2012). Future interventions should address communication in the relationship between the caregiver and healthcare professionals, particularly regarding caregivers' ability to access medical information about rehabilitation and palliative care (Aoun et al., 2012). Difficulty in obtaining satisfying information is one of the major sources of caregiver stress (Aoun et al., 2012). Thus, this type of intervention may empower caregivers as the users of health care services and improve their health literacy.

In the same vein, future research and applications need to address the multiple barriers to implementing evidence-based interventions in real-life practice settings (Northouse et al., 2012). The barriers include a lack of awareness of caregiver needs among healthcare professionals, a lack of training for healthcare professionals on how to intervene with caregivers, as well as organizational, time-related, and financial barriers in healthcare systems (Northouse et al., 2012). The recognition of the importance of interventions for caregivers should be reflected in best practice recommendations.

This brings us to possibly the most important change that needs to be made: establishing evidence-based best practice recommendations for caregivers. A proposal providing care to cancer caregivers in healthcare practice settings was issued by Northouse et al. (2012), suggesting t three core areas: assessment, education, and resource and services. Assessment includes evaluation of the caregiver's willingness and ability to provide care (physical, emotional, and cognitive ability), as well as measurement of knowledge and skill levels. Education accounts for caregiver tasks, stress management, promotion of caregivers' health (including nutrition and exercise), and disease prevention (e.g., screening). The resources and services component refers to the evaluation of available, utilized, and needed resources for the caregiver from primary care provider and the availability of social support (either in groups or by telephone or web) and respite care (Northouse et al., 2012).

Conclusion

Despite the limitations of the studies, there is a growing body of evidence indicating that interventions for caregivers reduce depression, stress, and anxiety, improve quality of life and physical functioning, and enhance competence and mastery. The evidence base suggests that effective interventions address caregiving-related skills, knowledge, abilities of coping with daily stress, and communication with patient. However, as more and more people will require caregiving in the near future, it behooves us to study what components of interventions are effective for which populations of caregivers at which points of the illness trajectory. This is a complex request, but an essential one.

References

Abell, N. (2001). Assessing willingness to care for persons with AIDS: Validation of a new measure. *Research on Social Work Practice, 11*(1), 118–130. doi: 10.1177/104973150101100108

Abraham, C., Johnson, B. J., de Bruin, M., & Luszczynska, A. (2014). Enhancing reporting of behavior change intervention evaluations. *Journal of Acquired Immune Deficiency Syndromes, 66,* 293–299. doi:10.1097/QAI.0000000000000231

Abraído-Lanza, A.F., & Revenson, T.A. (2006). Illness intrusion and psychological adjustment to rheumatic diseases: A social identity framework. *Arthritis and Rheumatism: Arthritis Care & Research, 55*(2), 224–232. doi:10.1002/art.21849

Addington-Hall, J. M., MacDonald, L. D., Anderson, H. R., Chamberlain, J., Freeling, P., Bland, J. M., & Raftery, J. (1992). Randomised controlled trial of effects of coordinating care for terminally ill cancer patients. *British Medical Journal, 305*(6865), 1317–1322. doi:10.1136/bmj.305.6865.1317

Adelman, R. D., Tmanova, L. L., Delgado, D., Dion, S., & Lachs, M. S. (2014). Caregiver burden: A clinical review. *The Journal of the American Medical Association, 311,* 1052–1060. doi:10.1001/jama.2014.304

Ahmad, W. I. U. (2000). Introduction. In W. I. U. Ahmad (Ed.), *Ethnicity, disability and chronic illness* (pp. 1–11). Buckingham, UK: Open University Press.

Al-Janabi, H., Frew, E., Brouwer, W., Rappange, D., & Van Exel, J. (2010). The inclusion of positive aspects of caring in the Caregiver Strain Index: Tests of feasibility and validity. *International Journal of Nursing Studies, 47*(8), 984–993. doi:10.1016/j.ijnurstu.2009.12.015

An, A. R., Lee, J., Yun, Y. H., & Heo, D. S. (2014). Terminal cancer patients' and their primary caregivers' attitudes toward hospice/palliative care and their effects on actual utilization: A prospective cohort study. *Palliative Medicine, 28*(7), 976–985. doi:10.1177/0269216314531312

Aneshensel, C. S., Pearlin, L. I., Mullan, J. T., Zarit, S. H., & Whitlatch, C. J. (1995). *Profiles in caregiving: The unexpected career.* San Diego, CA: Academic Press.

Antonovsky, A. (1993). The structure and properties of the sense of coherence scale. *Social Science & Medicine, 36*, 725–733. doi:10.1016/0277-9536(93)90033-Z

Aoun, S. M., Bentley, B., Funk, L., Toye, C., Grande, G., & Stajduhar, K. J. (2012). A 10-year literature review of family caregiving for motor neuron disease: Moving from caregiver burden studies to palliative care interventions. *Palliative Medicine, 27*, 437–446. doi:10.1177/0269216312455729

Aranda, M. P., & Knight, B. G. (1997). The influence of ethnicity and culture on the caregiver stress and coping process: A sociocultural review and analysis. *The Gerontologist, 37*(3), 342–254. doi:10.1093/geront/37.3.342

Arenstein, L. M., & Brown, R. T. (2014). Psychological aspects of caregiving. In R. C. Talley & S. S. Travis (Eds.), *Multidisciplinary coordinated caregiving: Research, practice, policy* (pp. 69–82). New York: Springer.

Arksey, H., & Moree, M. (2008). Supporting working carers: Do policies in England and the Netherlands reflect "doualia rights"? *Health & Social Care in the Community, 16*(6), 649–657. doi:10.1111/j.1365-2524.2008.00791.x

Badr, H., Carmack, C. L., Kashy, D. A., Cristofanilli, M., & Revenson, T. A. (2010). Dyadic coping in metastatic breast cancer. *Health Psychology, 29*(2), 169–180. doi:10.1037/a0018165

Badr, H., Gupta, V., Sikora, A., & Posner, M. (2014). Psychological distress in patients and caregivers over the course of radiotherapy for head and neck cancer. *Oral Oncology, 50*(10), 1005–1011. doi:10.1016/j.oraloncology.2014.07.003

Badr, H., & Krebs, P. (2013). A systematic review and meta-analysis of psychosocial interventions for couples coping with cancer. *Psycho-Oncology, 22*(8), 1688–1704. doi:10.1002/pon.3200

Badr, H., & Taylor, C. L. C. (2009). Sexual dysfunction and spousal communication in couples coping with prostate cancer. *Psycho-Oncology, 18*(7), 735–746. doi:10.1002/pon.1449

Bakas, T., & Champion, V. (1999). Development and psychometric testing of the Bakas Caregiving Outcomes Scale. *Nursing Research, 48*(5), 250–259. doi:10.1097/00006199-199909000-00005

Bakas, T., Champion, V., Perkins, S. M., Farran, C. J., & Williams, L. S. (2006). Psychometric testing of the revised 15-item Bakas Caregiving Outcomes Scale. *Nursing Research, 55*(5), 346–355. doi:10.1097/00006199-200609000-00007

Baker, K. L., Robertson, N., & Connelly, D. (2010). Men caring for wives or partners with dementia: Masculinity, strain and gain. *Aging & Mental Health, 14*(3), 319–327. doi:10.1080/13607860903228788

Bastawrous, M., Gignac, M. A., Kapral, M. K., & Cameron, J. I. (2014). Factors that contribute to adult children caregivers' well-being: A scoping review. *Health & Social Care in the Community, 1*, 1–18. doi:10.1111/hsc.12144

Batson, C. D. (1991). *The altruism question: Toward a social psychological answer*. Hillsdale, NJ: Lawrence Erlbaum Associates

Beeber, A. S., & Zimmerman, S. (2012). Adapting the Family Management Style Framework (FMSF) for families caring for older adults with dementia. *Journal of Family Nursing, 18*(1), 123–145. doi:10.1177/1074840711427144

Berg, C. A., & Upchurch, R. (2007). A developmental-contextual model of couples coping with chronic illness across the adult life span. *Psychological Bulletin, 133*(6), 920–954. doi:10.1037/0033-2909.133.6.920

Berg, C. A., Wiebe, D. J., Butner, J., Bloor, L., Bradstreet, C., Upchurch, R., Hayes, J, Stephenson, R., Nail, L., & Patton, G. (2008). Collaborative coping and daily mood in couples dealing with prostate cancer. *Psychology & Aging, 23*(3), 505–516. doi:10.1037/a0012687

Berge, J. M., Patterson, J. M., & Rueter, M. (2006). Marital satisfaction and mental health of couples with children with chronic health conditions. *Families, Systems, & Health, 24*(3), 267. doi:10.1037/1091-7527.24.3.267

Beisecker, A. E., Wright, L. J., Chrisman, S. K., & Ashworth, J. (1996). Family caregiver perceptions of benefits and barriers to the use of adult day care for individuals with Alzheimer's disease. *Research on Aging, 18*(4), 430–450. doi:10.1177/0164027596184003

Bialon, L. N., & Coke, S. (2012). A study on caregiver burden stressors, challenges, and possible solutions. *American Journal of Hospice & Palliative Medicine, 29*(3), 210–218. doi:10.1177/1049909111416494

Blake, H., Lincoln, N. B., & Clarke, D. D. (2003). Caregiver strain in spouses of stroke patients. *Clinical Rehabilitation, 17*(3), 312–317. doi:10.1191/0269215503cr6130a

Blum, K., & Sherman, D. W. (2010). Understanding the experience of caregivers: A focus on transitions. *Seminars in Oncology Nursing, 26*(4), 243–258. doi:10.1016/j.soncn.2010.08.005

Boehmer, U., & Clark, J. (2001). Communication about prostate cancer between men and their wives. *Journal of Family Practice, 50*(3), 226–231.

Boerner, K., Schulz, R., & Horowitz, A. (2004). Positive aspects of caregiving and adaptation to bereavement. *Psychology & Aging, 19*(4), 668–675. doi:10.1037/0882-7974.19.4.668

Bond, M. J., Clark, M. S., & Davies, S. (2003). The quality of life of spouse dementia caregivers: Changes associated with yielding to formal care and widowhood. *Social Science & Medicine, 57*(12), 2385–2395. doi:10.1016/S0277-9536(03)00133-3

Bookwala, J., & Schulz, R. (1998). The role of neuroticism and mastery in spouse caregivers' assessment of and response to a contextual stressor. *The Journals of Gerontology Series B: Psychological Sciences and Social Sciences of Gerontology, 53*, 155–164. doi:10.1093/geronb/53B.3.P155

Bosman, L. (2014). *Naupaka*. The Netherlands: De Vrije Uitgevers.

Bowlby, J. (1973). *Attachment and loss, vol. 2: Separation*. New York: Basic Books.

Bowlby, J. (1982). *Attachment and loss: vol. 1: Attachment*, 2nd edition. New York: Basic Books.

Bowlby, J. (1988). *A secure base: Parent-child attachment and healthy human development*. New York: Basic Books.

Brandão, T., Schulz, M. S., & Matos, P. M. (2014). Psychological intervention with couples coping with breast cancer: A systematic review. *Psychology & Health, 29*(5), 491–516. doi:10.1080/08870446.2013.859257

Braun, M., Mikulincer, M., Rydall, A., Walsh, A., & Rodin, G. (2007). Hidden morbidity in cancer: Spouse caregivers. *Journal of Clinical Oncology, 25*, 4829–2834. doi:10.1200/JCO.2006.10.0909

Braun, M., Mura, K., Peter-Wight, M., Hornung, R., & Scholz, U. (2010). Toward a better understanding of psychological well-being in dementia caregivers: The link between marital communication and depression. *Family Process, 49*(2), 185–203. doi:10.1111/j.1545-5300.2010.01317.x

Brodaty, H., & Donkin, M. (2009). Family caregivers of people with dementia. *Dialogues in Clinical Neuroscience, 11*(2), 217.

Brody, E. M. (1985). Parent care as a normative family stress. *The Gerontologist, 25*(1), 19–29. doi:10.1093/geront/25.1.19

Brody, E. M., Hoffman, C., Kleban, M. H., & Schoonover, C. B. (1988). Parent care and sibling relationships: Perceptions of caregiving daughters and their local siblings. *The Gerontologist, 30*, 25–34. doi:10.1093/geront/29.4.529

Brouwer, W. B. F., Van Exel, N. J. A., Van den Berg, B., Van den Bos, G. A., & Koopmanschap, M. A. (2005). Process utility from providing informal care: The benefit of caring. *Health Policy, 74*(1), 85–99. doi:10.1016/j.healthpol.2004.12.008

Brouwer, W. B. F., Van Exel, N. J. A., Van Gorp, B., & Redekop, W. K. (2006). The CarerQol instrument: A new instrument to measure care-related quality of life of informal caregivers for use in economic evaluations. *Quality of Life Research, 15*(6), 1005–1021. doi:10.1007/s11136-005-5994-6

Brown, S. L., Smith, D. M., Schulz, R., Kabeto, M. U., Ubel, P. A., Poulin, M., Yi, J., Kim, C., & Langa, K. M. (2009). Caregiving behavior is associated with decreased mortality risk. *Psychological Science, 20*(4), 488–494. doi:10.1111/j.1467-9280.2009.02323.x

Burridge, L., Winch, S., & Clavarino, A. (2007). Reluctance to care: A systematic review and development of a conceptual framework. *Cancer Nursing, 30*(2), 9–19. doi:10.1097/01.NCC.0000265298.17394.e0

Calasanti, T., & King, N. (2007). Taking "women's work" "like a man": Husbands' experiences of care work. *The Gerontologist, 47*, 516–527. doi:10.1093/geront/47.4.516

Carers UK (2014). State of Caring Survey, London: Carers UK Census (2001). Office for National Statistics; General Register Office for Scotland. http://www.statistics.gov.uk. Retrieved July 15, 2015.

Carnelley, K. B., Pietromonaco, P. R., & Jaffe, K. (1996). Attachment, caregiving, and relationship functioning in couples: Effects of self and partner. *Personal Relationships, 3*, 257–278. doi:10.1111/j.1475-6811.1996.tb00116.x

Carver, C. S., & Scheier, M. (1998). *On the self-regulation of behavior.* New York: Cambridge University Press.

Carver, C. S., Scheier, M. F., Miller, C. J., & Fulford, D. (2009). Optimism. In S. J. Lopez & C. R. Snyder (Eds.), *The Oxford handbook of positive psychology* (pp. 303–311). New York: Oxford University Press. doi:10.1093/oxfordhb/9780195398694.001.0001

Cary, M. S., Rubright, J. D., Grill, J. D., & Karlawish, J. (2015). Why are spousal caregivers more prevalent than nonspousal caregivers as study partners in AD dementia clinical trials? *Alzheimer Disease & Associated Disorders, 29*(1), 70–74. doi:10.1097/WAD.0000000000000047

Cassidy, T., Mclaughlin, M., & Giles, M. (2015). Applying a resource model of stress to the cancer caregiver experience. *Clinical Nursing Studies, 3*, 59–66. doi:10.5430/cns.v3n2p59

Chappell, N. L., Dujela, C., & Smith, A. (2014). Caregiver well-being intersections of relationship and gender. *Research on Aging, 37*(6), 623–645. doi:10.1177/0164027514549258

Cheng, H. Y., Chair, S. Y., & Chau, J. P. C. (2014). The effectiveness of psychosocial interventions for stroke family caregivers and stroke survivors: A systematic review and meta-analysis. *Patient Education & Counseling, 95*, 30–44. doi:10.1016/j.pec.2014.01.005

Chi, N-C., & Demiris, G. (2015). A systematic review of telehealth tools and interventions to support family caregivers. *Journal of Telemedicine & Telecare, 21*, 37–44. doi:10.1177/1357633X14562734

Chindaprasirt, J., Limpawattana, P., Pakkaratho, P., Wirasorn, K., Sookprasert, A., Kongbunkiat, K., & Sawanyawisuth, K. (2014). Burdens among caregivers of older adults with advanced cancer and risk factors. *Asian Pacific Journal of Cancer Prevention, 15*(4), 1643–1648. doi.org/10.7314/APJCP.2014.15.4.1643

Christakis, N. A., & Iwashyna, T. J. (2003). The health impact of health care on families: A matched cohort study of hospice use by decedents and mortality outcomes in surviving, widowed spouses. *Social Science & Medicine, 57*(3), 465–475. doi:10.1016/S0277-9536(02)00370-2

Chun, C., Moos, R. H., & Cronkite, R. C. (2006). CULTURE: A fundamental context for the stress and coping paradigm. In P. T. P. Wong & L. C. J. Wong (Eds.), *Handbook of multicultural perspectives on stress and coping, international and cultural psychology* (pp. 29–53). New York: Springer.

Chun, M., Knight, B. G., & Youn, G. (2007). Differences in stress and coping models of emotional distress among Korean, Korean-American and White-American caregivers. *Aging & Mental Health, 11*(1), 20–29. doi:10.1080/13607860600736232

Chung, M. L., Moser, D. K., Lennie, T. A., & Rayens, M. K. (2009). The effects of depressive symptoms and anxiety on quality of life in patients with heart failure and their spouses: Testing dyadic dynamics using Actor–Partner Interdependence Model. *Journal of Psychosomatic Research, 67*(1), 29–35. doi:10.1016/j.jpsychores.2009.01.009

Clark, L. M., & Hartman, M. (1996). Effects of hardiness and appraisal on the psychological distress and physical health of caregivers to elderly relatives. *Research on Aging, 18*(4), 379–401. doi:10.1177/0164027596184001

Clark, M. S., & Monin, J. K. (2006). Giving and receiving communal responsiveness as love. In R. J. Sternberg & K. Weis (Eds.), *The new psychology of love* (pp. 200–221). New Haven, CT: Yale University Press.

Cohen, O., Birnbaum, G. E., Meyuchas, R., Levinger, Z., Florian, V., & Mikulincer, M. (2005). Attachment orientations and spouse support in adults with type 2 diabetes. *Psychology, Health & Medicine, 10*, 161–165. doi:10.1080/13548500420000326575

Coon, D. W., Rubert, M., Solano, N., Mausbach, B., Kraemer, H., Arguelles, T., Haley, W. E., Thompson, L. W., & Gallagher-Thompson, D. (2004). Well-being, appraisal, and coping in Latina and Caucasian female dementia caregivers: Findings from the REACH study. *Aging & Mental Health, 8*(4), 330–345. doi:10.1080/13607860410001709683

Cooper, C., Katona, C., Orrell, M., & Livingston, G. (2008). Coping strategies, anxiety and depression in caregivers of people with Alzheimer's disease. *International Journal of Geriatric Psychiatry, 23*(9), 929–936. doi: 10.1002/gps.2007

Coristine, M., Crooks, D., Grunfeld, E., Stonebridge, C., & Christie, A. (2003). Caregiving for women with advanced breast cancer. *Psycho-Oncology, 12*(7), 709–719. doi:10.1002/pon.696

Corry, M., While, A., Neenan, K., & Smith, V. (2015). A systematic review of systematic reviews on interventions for caregivers of people with chronic conditions. *Journal of Advanced Nursing, 71*, 718–734. doi:10.1111/jan.12523

Cotrell, V., & Engel, R. J. (1999). The role of secondary supports in mediating formal services to dementia caregivers. *Journal of Gerontological Social Work, 30*(3–4), 117–132. doi:10.1300/J083v30n03_10

Cousino, M. K., & Hazen, R. A. (2013). Parenting stress among caregivers of children with chronic illness: A systematic review. *Journal of Pediatric Psychology, 38*(8), 809–828. doi:10.1093/jpepsy/jst049

Covinsky, K. E., Newcomer, R., Fox, P., Wood, J., Sands, L., Dane, K., & Yaffe, K. (2003). Patient and caregiver characteristics associated with depression in caregivers of patients with dementia. *Journal of General Internal Medicine, 18*(12), 1006–1014. doi:10.1111/j.1525-1497.2003.30103.x

Coyne, J. C., & Smith, D. A. (1991). Couples coping with a myocardial infarction: A contextual perspective on wives' distress. *Journal of Personality and Social Psychology, 61*(3), 404. doi:10.1037/0022

Dagan, M., & Hagedoorn, M. (2014). Response rates in studies of couples coping with cancer: A systematic review. *Health Psychology, 33*(8), 845–852. doi:10.1037/hea0000013

Dagan, M., Sanderman, R., Hoff, C., Meijerink, W. J. H. J., Baas, P. C., van Haastert, M., & Hagedoorn, M. (2014). The interplay between partners' responsiveness and patients' need for emotional expression in couples coping with cancer. *Journal of Behavioral Medicine, 37*(5), 828–838. doi:10.1007/s10865-013-9543-4

Dagan, M., Sanderman, R., Schokker, M. C., Wiggers, T., Baas, P. C., van Haastert, M., & Hagedoorn, M. (2011). Spousal support and changes in distress over time in couples coping with cancer: The role of personal control. *Journal of Family Psychology, 25*(2), 310–318. doi:10.1037/a0022887

De Vugt, M. E., Stevens, F., Aalten, P., Lousberg, R., Jaspers, N., Winkens, I., Jolles, J., & Verhey, F. R. J. (2004). Do caregiver management strategies influence patient behaviour in dementia? *International Journal of Geriatric Psychiatry, 19*, 85–92. doi:10.1002/gps.1041

Deeken, J. F., Taylor, K. L., Mangan, P., Yabroff, K. R., & Ingham, J. M. (2003). Care for the caregivers: A review of self-report instruments developed to measure the burden, needs, and quality of life of informal caregivers. *Journal of Pain and Symptom Management, 26*(4), 922–953. doi:10.1016/S0885-3924(03)00327-0

Dekel, R., Vilchinsky, N., Liberman, G., Leibowitz, M., Khaskia, A., & Mosseri, M. (2014). Marital satisfaction and depression among couples following men's acute coronary syndrome: Testing dyadic dynamics in a longitudinal design. *British Journal of Health Psychology, 19*(2), 347–362. doi:10.1111/bjhp.12042

Denby, R. W., Brinson, J. A., Cross, C. L., & Bowmer, A. (2014). Male kinship caregivers: Do they differ from their female counterparts? *Children & Youth Services Review, 46*, 248–256. doi:10.1016/j.childyouth.2014.09.003

Denton, M., Prus, S., & Walters, V. (2004). Gender differences in health: A Canadian study of the psychosocial, structural and behavioural determinants of health. *Social Science & Medicine, 58*(12), 2585–2600. doi:10.1016/j.socscimed.2003.09.008

Dettinger, E., & Clarkberg, M. (2002). Informal caregiving and retirement timing among men and women: Gender and caregiving relationships in late midlife. *Journal of Family Issues, 23*(7), 857–879. doi:10.1177/019251302236598

Diefenbach, M. A., Badr, H. Revenson, T. A., Herrera, P. C., Knauer, C., Tewari, A., & Hall, S. J. (2015, April). Brief intervention to improve QOL & couple functioning after prostate surgery. In M. A. Diefenbach (Chair), *Advances in dyadic research: Exploring novel delivery formats, intervention targets and health behaviors*. Symposium presented at the Annual Meeting of the Society for Behavioral Medicine, San Antonio, TX.

Dilworth-Anderson, P., Williams, I. C., & Gibson, B. E. (2002). Issues of race, ethnicity, and culture in caregiving research: A 20-year review (1980–2000). *The Gerontologist, 42*(2), 237–272. doi:10.1093/geront/42.2.237

Diwan, S., Hougham, G. W., & Sachs, G. A. (2004). Strain experienced by caregivers of dementia patients receiving palliative care: Findings from the Palliative Excellence in Alzheimer Care Efforts (PEACE) Program. *Journal of Palliative Medicine, 7*(6), 797–807. doi:10.1089/jpm.2004.7.797

Dooley, K. W., Shaffer, D. R., Lance, C. E., & Williamson, G. M. (2007). Informal care can be better than adequate: Development and evaluation of the Exemplary Care Scale. *Rehabilitation Psychology, 52*(4), 359–369. doi:10.1037/0090-5550.52.4.359

Douglass, L. G. (1997). Reciprocal support in the context of cancer: Perspectives of the patient and spouse. *Oncology Nursing Forum, 24*(9), 1529–1536.

Dracup, K., Evangelista, L. S., Doering, L., Tullman, D., Moser, D. K., & Hamilton, M. (2004). Emotional well-being in spouses of patients with advanced heart failure. *Heart & Lung, 33*, 354–361. doi:10.1016/j.hrtlng.2004.06.003

Duggleby, W., Holtslander, L., Kylma, J., Duncan, V., Hammond, C., & Williams, A. (2010). Metasynthesis of the hope experience of family caregivers of persons with chronic illness. *Qualitative Health Research, 20*(2), 148–158. doi:10.1177/1049732309358329

Engel, G. L. (1977). The need for a new medical model: A challenge for biomedicine. *Science, 196*, 129–136. doi:10.1037/h0089260

Epiphaniou, E., Hamilton, D., Bridger, S., Robinson, V., Rob, G., Beynon, T., Harding, R. (2012). Adjusting to the caregiving role: The importance of coping and support. *International Journal of Palliative Nursing, 18*(11), 541–545. doi:10.12968/ijpn.2012.18.11.541

Etters, L., Goodall, D., & Harrison, B. E. (2008). Caregiver burden among dementia patient caregivers: A review of the literature. *Journal of the American Academy of Nurse Practitioners, 20*(8), 423–428. doi:10.1111/j.1745-7599.2008.00342.x

Esplen, E. (2009) *Gender and care: Overview report*. UK: Institute of Development Studies.

Evans, B. C., Coon, D. W., & Belyea, M. J. (2014). Worry among Mexican American caregivers of community-dwelling elders. *Hispanic Journal of Behavioral Sciences, 36*(3), 344–365. doi:10.1177/0739986314536684

Evercare and the National Alliance for Caregiving (2006). A close-up look at the health risks of caring for a loved one caregivers in decline – Report of findings. Minnetonka, MN: Evercare Health Plans. http://www.caregiving.org/data/Caregivers%20in%20Decline%20Study-FINAL-lowres.pdf. Retrieved June 26, 2015.

Family Caregiver Alliance (2006). Caregiver assessment: principles, guidelines and strategies for change: Report from a National Consensus Development Conference. https://caregiver.org/sites/caregiver.org/files/pdfs/v1_consensus.pdf. Retrieved July 15, 2015.

Family Caregiver Alliance (2015). Women and caregiving: Facts and figures. https://caregiver.org/women-and-caregiving-facts-and-figures. Retrieved July 2, 2015.

Feeney, B. C., & Collins, N. L. (2001). Predictors of caregiving in adult intimate relationships: An attachment theoretical perspective. *Journal of Personality & Social Psychology, 80*, 972–994. doi:10.1037/0022-3514.80.6.972

Feeney, J. A., & Ryan, S. M. (1994). Attachment style and affect regulation: Relationships with health behavior and family experiences of illness in a student sample. *Health Psychology, 13*, 334–345. doi:10.1037/0278-6133.13.4.334

Feinberg, L. Reinhard, S. C., Houser, A., & Choula, R. (2011). Valuing the invaluable: 2011 update: The growing contributions and Costs of Family Caregiving. AARP Policy Institute. http://assets.aarp.org/rgcenter/ppi/ltc/fs229-ltc.pdf. Retrieved July 2, 2015.

Ferguson, E. (2013). Personality is of central concern to understand health: Towards a theoretical model for health psychology. *Health Psychology Review, 7*, 32–70. doi:10.1080/17437199.2010.547985

Ferrario, S. R., Baiardi, P., & Zotti, A. M. (2004). Update on the family strain questionnaire: A tool for the general screening of caregiving-related problems. *Quality of Life Research, 13*(8), 1425–1434. doi:10.1023/B:QURE.0000040795.78742.72

Fianco, A., Sartori, R. D. G., Negri, L., Lorini, S., Valle, G., & Fave, A. D. (2015). The relationship between burden and well-being among caregivers of Italian people diagnosed with severe neuromotor and cognitive disorders. *Research in Developmental Disabilities, 39*, 43–54. doi:10.1016/j.ridd.2015.01.006

Figueiredo, D., Gabriel, R., Jacome, C., & Marques, A. (2013). Caring for people with early and advanced chronic obstructive pulmonary disease: How do family carers cope? *Journal of Clinical Nursing, 23*(1–2), 211–220. doi:10.1111/jocn.12363

Fletcher, B. S., Miaskowski, C., Given, B., & Schumacher, K. (2012). The cancer family caregiving experience: An updated and expanded conceptual model. *European Journal of Oncology Nursing, 16*(4), 387–398. doi:10.1016/j.ejon.2011.09.001

Folkman, S. (1984). Personal control and stress and coping processes: A theoretical analysis. *Journal of Personality & Social Psychology, 46*, 839–852. doi: 10.1037/0022-3514.46.4.839

Forster, A., Dickerson, J., Melbourn, A., Steadman, J., Wittink, M., Young, J., Kalra, L., & Farrin, A. (2015). The development and implementation of the structured training programme for caregivers of inpatients after stroke (TRACS) intervention: The London Stroke Carers Training. *Clinical Rehabilitation, 29*, 211–220. doi:10.1177/0269215514543334

Fox, S., & Brenner, J. (2012). Family caregivers online. Washington, DC: Pew Research Center's Internet & American Life Project. http://pewinternet.org/Reports/2012/Caregivers-online.aspx. Retrieved June 27, 2015.

Fredman, L., Cauley, J. A., Satterfield, S., Simonsick, E., Spencer, S. M., Ayonayon, H. N., & Harris, T. B. (2008). Caregiving, mortality, and mobility decline: The Health, Aging, and Body Composition (Health ABC) study. *Archives of Internal Medicine, 168*(19), 2154–2162. doi:10.1001/archinte.168.19.2154

Freedman, V. A., Cornman, J. C., & Carr, D. (2014). Is spousal caregiving associated with enhanced well-being? New evidence from the panel study of income dynamics. *The Journals of Gerontology*

Series B: Psychological Sciences and Social Sciences, 69(6), 861–869. doi:10.1093/geronb/gbu004

Friedman, H. S. (2011). Personality, disease, and self-healing. In H. S. Friedman (Ed.), *The Oxford handbook of health psychology* (pp. 215–240). New York: Oxford University Press. doi:10.1093/oxfordhb/9780195342819.013.0010

Friedemann, M. L., & Buckwalter, K. C. (2014). Family caregiver role and burden related to gender and family relationships. *Journal of Family Nursing, 2*(3), 313–336. doi:1074840714532715

Fritz, H. L. (2000). Gender-linked personality traits predict mental health and functional status following a first coronary event. *Health Psychology, 19*(5), 420–428. doi:10.1037/0278-6133.19.5.420

Funk, L. M., Chappell, N. L., & Liu, G. (2013). Associations between filial responsibility and caregiver well-being: Are there differences by cultural group? *Research on Aging, 35*(1), 78–95. doi:10.1177/0164027511422450

Gallagher-Thompson, D., Solano, N., Coon, D., & Areán, P. (2003). Recruitment and retention of Latino dementia family caregivers in intervention research: Issues to face, lessons to learn. *The Gerontologist, 43*(1) 45–51. doi:10.1093/geront/43.1.45

Gallant, M. P., & Connell, C. M. (2003). Neuroticism and depressive symptoms among spouse caregivers: Do health behaviors mediate this relationship? *Psychology & Aging, 18*, 587–592. doi:10.1037/0882-7974.18.3.587

Gallup Organization (2011). Most caregivers look after elderly parent; invest a lot of time. http://www.gallup.com/poll/148682/caregivers-look-elderly-parent-invest-lot-time.aspx> July 28, 2011. Retrieved June 26, 2015.

Gaugler, J. E., Eppinger, A., King, J., Sandberg, T., & Regine, W. F. (2013). Coping and its effects on cancer caregiving. *Supportive Care in Cancer, 21*(2), 385–395. doi:10.1007/s00520-012-1525-5

Gaugler, J. E., Kane, R. L., & Newcome, R. (2005). The longitudinal effects of early behavior problems in the dementia caregiving career. *Psychology & Aging, 20*(1), 100–116. doi:10.1037/0882-7974.20.1.100

Gaugler, J. E., Zarit, S. H., & Pearlin, L. I. (2003). The onset of dementia caregiving and its longitudinal implications. *Psychology & Aging, 18*, 171–180. doi:10.1037/0882-7974.18.2.171

Gaynor, S. E. (1990). The long haul: The effects of home care on caregivers. *Image: The Journal of Nursing Scholarship, 22*(4), 208–212. doi:10.1111/j.1547-5069.1990.tb00215.x

Gemmill, R., & Cooke, L. (2011). Informal caregivers of hematopoietic cell transplant patients: A review and recommendations for interventions and research. *Cancer Nursing, 34*, 13–21. doi:10.1097/NCC.0b013e31820a592d

Gerstel, N., & Gallagher, S. K. (2001). Men's caregiving: Gender and the contingent character of care. *Gender & Society, 15*(2), 197–217. doi:10.1177/089124301015002003

Gilligan, C. (1982). *In a different voice*. Cambridge, MA: Harvard University Press.

Giunta, N., Chow, J., Scharlach, A. E., & Dal Santo, T. S. (2004). Racial and ethnic differences in family caregiving in California. *Journal of Human Behavior in the Social Environment, 9*(4), 85–109. doi:10.1300/J137v09n04_05

Given, C. W., Given, B., Stommel, M., Collins, C., King, S., & Franklin, S. (1992). The caregiver reaction assessment (CRA) for caregivers to persons with chronic physical and mental impairments. *Research in Nursing & Health, 15*(4), 271–283. doi:10.1002/nur.4770150406

Given, B. A., Sherwood, P., & Given, C. W. (2011). Support for caregivers of cancer patients: Transition after active treatment. *Cancer Epidemiology Biomarkers & Prevention, 20*(10), 2015–2021. doi:10.1158/1055-9965.EPI-11-0611

Goins, R. T., Spencer, S. M., McGuire L. C., Goldberg, J., Wen, Y., & Henderson, J. A. (2011). Adult caregiving among American Indians: The role of cultural factors. *The Gerontologist, 51*(3), 310–320. doi:10.1093/geront/gnq101

Gonzalez-Abraldes, I., Millan-Calenti, J. C., Lorenzo-Lopez, L., & Maseda, A. (2013) The influence of neuroticism and extraversion on the perceived burden of dementia caregivers: An exploratory study. *Archives of Gerontology & Geriatrics, 56*, 91–95. doi:10.1016/j.archger.2012.07.011

Goy, E. R. (2012). Review: Supportive interventions may improve short-term psychological distress in informal caregivers of patients at the end of life. *Evidence Based Metal Health, 15,* 21. doi:10.1136/ebmental-2011-100350

Gross, J. J., & John, O. P. (2003). Individual differences in two emotion regulation processes: Implications for affect, relationships, and well-being. *Journal of Personality and Social Psychology, 85*(2), 348–362. doi:10.1037/0022-3514.85.2.348

Grov, E. K., Fosså, S. D., Tønnessen, A., & Dahl, A. A. (2006). The caregiver reaction assessment: Psychometrics, and temporal stability in primary caregivers of Norwegian cancer patients in late palliative phase. *Psycho-Oncology, 15*(6), 517–527. doi:10.1002/pon.987

Grunfeld, E., Coyle, D., Whelan, T., Clinch, J., Reyno, L., Earle, C. C., Willan, A., Viola, R., Coristine, M., Janz, T., & Glossop, R. (2004). Family caregiver burden: Results of a longitudinal study of breast cancer patients and their principal caregivers. *Canadian Medical Association Journal, 170*(12), 1795–1801. doi:10.1503/cmaj.1031205

Gujral, U. P., Pradeepa, R., Weber, M. B., Narayan, K. M., & Mohan, V. (2013). Type 2 diabetes in South Asians: Similarities and differences with white Caucasian and other populations. *Annals of the New York Academy of Sciences, 1281*(1), 51–63. doi:10.1111/j.1749-6632.2012.06838.x

Gupta, R., & Pillai, V. K. (2002). Elder care giving in South Asian families: Implications for social service. *Journal of Comparative Family Studies, 33*(4), 565–576.

Gupta, R., Rowe, N., & Pillai, V. K. (2009). Perceived caregiver burden in India: Implications for social services. *Affilia: Journal of Women & Social Work, 24*(1), 69–79. doi:10.1177/0886109908326998

Hafstrom, J. L., & Schram, V. R. (1984). Chronic illness in couples: Selected characteristics, including wife's satisfaction with and perception of marital relationships. *Family Relations, 33*, 195–203. doi: 10.2307/584605

Hagedoorn, M., Buunk, B. P., Kuijer, R. G., Wobbes, T., & Sanderman, R. (2000). Couples dealing with cancer: Role and gender differences regarding psychological distress and quality of life. *Psycho-Oncology, 9*(3), 232–242. doi:10.1002/1099-1611(200005/06)9:3<232::AID-PON458>3.0.CO;2-J

Hagedoorn, M., Dagan, M., Puterman, E., Hoff, C., Meijerink, W. J. H. J., DeLongis, A., & Sanderman, R. (2011). Relationship satisfaction in couples confronted with colorectal cancer: The interplay of past and current spousal support. *Journal of Behavioral Medicine, 34*(4), 288–297. doi:10.1007/s10865-010-9311-7

Hagedoorn, M., Sanderman, R., Bolks, H. N., Tuinstra, J., & Coyne, J. C. (2008). Distress in couples coping with cancer: A meta-analysis and critical review of role and gender effects. *Psychological Bulletin, 134*(1), 1–30. doi:10.3322/caac.20081

Hagedoorn, M., Sanderman, R. Buunk, B. P., & Wobbes, T. (2002). Failing in spousal caregiving: The "identity-relevant stress" hypothesis to explain sex differences in caregiver distress. *British Journal of Health Psychology, 7*, 481–494. doi:10.1348/135910702320645435

Hagedoorn, M., Sanderman, R., Ranchor, A., Brilman, E., Kempen, G., & Ormel, J. (2001). Chronic disease in elderly couples – Are women more responsive to their spouses' health condition than men? *Journal of Psychosomatic Research, 51*(5), 693–696. doi:10.1016/S0022-3999(01)00279-3

Hagedoorn, M., Puterman, E., Sanderman, R., Wiggers, T., Baas, P. C., van Haastert, M., & DeLongis, A. (2011). Is self-disclosure in couples coping with cancer associated with improvement in depressive symptoms? *Health Psychology, 30*(6), 753–762. doi:10.1037/a0024374

Haines, K. J., Denehy, L., Skinner, E. H., Warrillow, S., & Berney, S. (2015). Psychosocial outcomes in informal caregivers of the critically ill: A systematic review. *Critical Care Medicine, 43*(5), 1112–1120. doi:10.1097/CCM.0000000000000865

Halm, M. A., & Bakas, T. (2007). Factors associated with caregiver depressive symptoms, outcomes, and perceived physical health after coronary artery bypass surgery. *Journal of Cardiovascular Nursing, 22*, 508–515. doi:10.1097/01.JCN.0000297388.21626.6c

Halm, M. A., Treat-Jacobson, D., Lindquist, R., & Savik, K. (2007). Caregiver burden and outcomes of caregiving of spouses of patients who undergo coronary artery bypass graft surgery. *Heart & Lung: The Journal of Acute and Critical Care, 36*(3), 170–187. doi:10.1016/j.hrtlng.2006.08.003

Han, Y., Hu, D., Liu, Y., Lu, C., Luo, Z., Zhao, J., Lopez, V., & Mao, J. (2014). Coping styles and social support among depressed Chinese family caregivers of patients with esophageal cancer. *European Journal of Oncology Nursing, 18*(6), 571–577. doi:10.1016/j.ejon.2014.07.002

Hansen, T., & Slasvold, B. (2015). Feeling the squeeze? The effects of combining work and informal caregiving on psychological well-being. *European Journal of Ageing, 12*, 51–60. doi:10.1007/s10433-014-0315-y

Harden, J. K., Sanda, M. G., Wei, J. T., Yarandi, H., Hembroff, L., Hardy, J., Northouse, L. L., & PROSTQA Consortium Study Group (2013a). Partners' long-term appraisal of their caregiving experience, marital satisfaction, sexual satisfaction, and quality of life 2 years after prostate cancer treatment. *Cancer Nursing, 36*(2), 104–113. doi:10.1097/NCC.0b013e3182567c03

Harden, J., Sanda, M. G., Wei, J. T., Yarandi, H. N., Hembroff, L., Hardy, J., & Northouse, L. (2013b). Survivorship after prostate cancer treatment: Spouses' quality of life at 36 months. *Oncology Nursing Forum, 40*(6), 567–573. doi:10.1188/13.ONF.567-573.

Harding, R., & Higginson, I. J. (2003). What is the best way to help caregivers in cancer and palliative care? A systematic literature review of interventions and their effectiveness. *Palliative Medicine, 17*, 63–74. doi:10.1191/0269216303pm667oa

Harding, R., List, S., Epiphaniou, E., & Jones, H. (2011). How can informal caregivers in cancer and palliative care be supported? An updated systematic literature review of interventions and their effectiveness. *Palliative Medicine, 26*, 7–22. doi:10.1177/0269216311409613

Harris, P. B. (2002). The voices of husbands and sons caring for a family member with dementia. In B. J. Kramer & E. H. Thompson (Eds.). *Men as caregivers: Theory, research, and service implications* (pp. 213–233). New York: Springer.

Hartmann, M., Baezner, E., Wild, B., Eisler, I. & Herzog, W. (2010). Effects of interventions involving the family in the treatment of adult patients with chronic physical diseases: A meta-analysis. *Psychotherapy & Psychosomatics, 79*, 136–148. doi:10.1159/000286958

Hasson-Ohayon, I., Goldzweig, G., Sela-Oren, T., Pizem, N., Bar-Sela, G., & Wolf, I. (2013). Attachment style, social support and finding meaning among spouses of colorectal cancer patients: Gender differences. *Palliative & Supportive Care, 13*, 527–535. doi:10.1017/S1478951513000242

Hays, J. C., Pieper, C. F., & Purser, J. L. (2003). Competing risk of household expansion or institutionalization in late life. *The Journals of Gerontology Series B: Psychological Sciences & Social Sciences, 58*(1), 11–20. doi:10.1093/geronb/58.1.S11

Hébert, R., Bravo, G., & Préville, M. (2000). Reliability, validity and reference values of the Zarit Burden Interview for assessing informal caregivers of community-dwelling older persons with dementia. *Canadian Journal on Aging, 19*(4), 494–507. doi:10.1017/S0714980800012484

Hebert, R. S., Dang, Q., & Schulz, R. (2006). Preparedness for the death of a loved one and mental health in bereaved caregivers of patients with dementia: Findings from the REACH study. *Journal of Palliative Medicine, 9*(3), 683–693. doi:10.1089/jpm.2006.9.683

Helgeson, V. S. (2012). Gender and health: A social psychological perspective. In A. Baum, T. A., Revenson, & J. E. Singer (Eds.). *Handbook of health psychology*, 2nd edition (pp. 518–537). New York: Psychology Press.

Helgeson, V. S. (1994). Relation of agency and communion to well-being: Evidence and potential explanations. *Psychological Bulletin, 116*, 412–428. doi:10.1037/0033-2909.116.3.412

Helgeson, V. S. (2003). Unmitigated communion and adjustment to breast cancer: Associations and explanations. *Journal of Applied Social Psychology, 33*(8), 1643–1661. doi:10.1111/j.1559-1816.2003.tb01967.x

Helgeson, V. S., & Fritz, H. (1998). A theory of unmitigated communion. *Personality & Social Psychology Review, 2*, 173–183. doi:10.1037/0022-3514.75.1.121

Helgeson, V. S., & Lepore, S. J. (2004). Quality of life following prostate cancer: The role of agency and unmitigated agency. *Journal of Applied Social Psychology, 34*(12), 2559–2585. doi:10.1111/j.1559-1816.2004.tb01992.x

Heller, P. L. (1976). Familism Scale: Revalidation and revision. *Journal of Marriage and the Family, 38*(3), 423–429. doi:10.2307/350410

Hickman, S. E., Cartwright, J. C., Nelson, C. A., & Knafl, K. (2012). Compassion and vigilance: Investigators' strategies to manage ethical concerns in palliative and end-of-life research. *Journal of Palliative Medicine, 15*(8), 880–889. doi:10.1089/jpm.2011.0515

Hiel, L., Beenackers, M. A., Renders, C. M., Robroek, S. J. W., Burdorf, A., & Croezen, S. (2015). Providing personal informal care to older European adults: Should we care about the caregivers' health? *Preventive Medicine, 70*, 64–68. doi:10.1016/j.ypmed.2014.10.028

Higginson, I. J., & Gao, W. (2008). Caregiver assessment of patients with advanced cancer: Concordance with patients, effect of burden and positivity. *Health Quality of Life Outcomes, 6*(1), 42. doi:10.1186/1477-7525-6-42

Hirschman, K., Joyce, C., James, B., Xie, S., & Karlawish, J. (2005). Do Alzheimer's disease patients want to participate in a treatment decision, and would their caregivers let them? *The Gerontologist, 45*(3), 381–388. doi: 10.1093/geront/45.3.381

Hirst, M. (2005). Carer distress: A prospective, population-based study. *Social Science & Medicine, 61*(3), 697–708. doi:10.1016/j.socscimed.2005.01.001

Hochschild, A. R. (1983). *The managed heart: The commercialization of human feeling.* Berkeley, CA: University of California Press.

Hoe, J., Katona, C., Orrell, M., & Livingston, G. (2007). Quality of life in dementia: Care recipient and caregiver perceptions of quality of life in dementia: The LASER-AD study. *International Journal of Geriatric Psychiatry, 22*(10), 1031–1036. doi:10.1002/gps.1786

Hollis-Sawyer, L. A. (2001). Adaptive, growth-oriented, and positive perceptions of mother-daughter elder caregiving relationships: A path-analytic investigation of predictors. *Journal of Women & Aging, 13*, 5–22. doi:10.1300/J074v13n03_02

Hook, J. L. (2010). Gender inequality in the welfare state: Sex segregation in housework, 1965–2003. *American Journal of Sociology, 115*, 1480–1523. doi:10.1086/651384

Hooker, K., Monahan, D. J., Bowman S. R, Frazier L. D., & Shifren, K. (1998). Personality counts for a lot: Predictors of mental and physical health of spouse caregivers in two disease groups. *The Journals of Gerontology Series B: Psychological Sciences and Social Sciences of Gerontology, 53*, 73–85. doi:10.1093/geronb/53B.2.P73

Hooker, K., Monahan, D., Shifren, K., & Hutchinson, C. (1992). Mental and physical health of spouse caregivers: The role of personality. *Psychology & Aging, 7*, 367–375. doi:10.1037/0882-7974.7.3.367

Horodyska, K., Luszczynska, A., van den Berg, M., Hendriksen, M., Roos, G., de Bourdeaudhuij, I., & Brug, J. (2015). Good practice characteristics of diet and physical activity interventions and policies: An umbrella review. *BMC Public Health 15*, 274–304. doi:10.1186/s12889-015-1354-9

Horsburgh, M. E., Laing, G. P., Beanlands, H. J., Meng, A. X., & Harwood, L. (2008). A new measure of "lay" care-giver activities. *Kidney International, 74*(2), 230–236. doi:10.1038/ki.2008.163

Hsu, H. C., & Shyu, Y. I. L. (2003). Implicit exchanges in family caregiving for frail elders in Taiwan. *Qualitative Health Research, 13*(8), 1078–1093. doi:10.1177/1049732303256370

Hudson, P. (2004). Positive aspects and challenges associated with caring for a dying relative at home. *International Journal of Palliative Nursing, 10*(2), 58–65. doi:10.12968/ijpn.2004.10.2.12454

Hughes, N., Locock, L., & Ziebland, S. (2103). Personal identity and the role of "carer" among relatives and friends of people with Multiple Sclerosis. *Social Science & Medicine, 96*, 78–85. doi:10.1016/j.socscimed.2013.07.023

Hung, S., Pickard, A. S., Witt, W. P., & Lambert, B. L. (2007). Pain and depression in caregivers affected their perception of pain in stroke patients. *Journal of Clinical Epidemiology, 60*(9), 963–970. doi:10.1016/j.jclinepi.2006.12.010

Hunstad, I., & Svindseth, M. F. (2011). Challenges in home-based palliative care in Norway: A qualitative study of spouses' experiences.

International Journal of Palliative Nursing, 17(7), 398–404. doi:10.12968/ijpn.2011.17.7.398

Hunt, D., & Smith, J. A. (2004). The personal experience of carers of stroke survivors: An interpretative phenomenological analysis. *Disability & Rehabilitation, 26*(16), 1000–1011. doi:10.1080/09638280410001702423

Jacobs, J. C., Laporte, A., Van Houtven, C. H., & Coyte, P. C. (2014). Caregiving intensity and retirement status in Canada. *Social Science & Medicine, 102*, 74–82. doi:10.1016/j.socscimed.2013.11.051

Jaracz, K., Grabowska-Fudala, B., Gorna, K., Jaracz, J., Moczko, J., & Kozubski, W. 2015)). Burden in caregivers of long-term stroke survivors: Prevalence and determinants at 6 months and 5 years after stroke. *Patient Education & Counseling, 98*, 1011–1016. doi:10.1016/j.pec.2015.04.008

Jin, L., Van Yperen, N. W., Sanderman, R., & Hagedoorn, M. (2010). Depressive symptoms and unmitigated communion in support providers. *European Journal of Personality, 24*, 56–70. doi:10.1002/per.741

Jylha, P., & Isometsa, E. (2006). The relationship of neuroticism and extraversion to symptoms of anxiety and depression in the general population. *Depression & Anxiety, 23*, 281–289. doi10.1002/da.20167

Kaltenbaugh, D. J., Klem, M. L., Hu, L., Turi, E., Haines, A. J., & Hagerty Lingler, J. (2015). Using web-based interventions to support caregivers of patients with cancer: A systematic review. *Oncology Nursing Forum, 42*, 156–164. doi:10.1188/15.ONF.156-164

Karantzas, G. C., Evans, L., & Foddy, M. (2010). The role of attachment in current and future parent caregiving. *The Journals of Gerontology Series B: Psychological Sciences and Social Sciences of Gerontology, 65*, 573–580.doi:10.1093/geronb/gbq047

Katbamna, S., Ahmad, W., Bhakta, P., Baker, R., & Parjker, G. (2004). Do they look after their own? Informal support for South Asian carers. *Health and Social Care in the Community, 12*(5), 398–406. doi:10.1111/j.1365-2524.2004.00509.x

Kayser, K., & Revenson, T. A. (in press). Including the cultural context in dyadic coping. In M. Falconier, A. Randall, & G. Bodenmann (Eds.), *International perspectives on dyadic coping*. New York: Wiley-Blackwell.

Kayser, K., & Scott, J. L. (2008). *Helping couples cope with women's cancers: An evidence-based approach for practitioners*. New York: Springer.

Kayser, K., Watson, L. E., & Andrade, J. T. (2007). Cancer as a "we-disease": Examining the process of coping from a relational perspective. *Family Systems & Health, 25,* 404–418. doi.org/10.1037/1091-7527.25.4.404

Keefe, F. J., Ahles, T. A., Porter, L. S., Sutton, L. M., McBride, C. M., Pope, M. S., & Baucom, D. H. (2003). The self-efficacy of family caregivers for helping cancer patients manage pain at end-of-life. *Pain, 103,* 157–162. doi:10.1016/S0304-3959(02)00448-7

Kelleher, D., & Hillier, S. (1996). *Researching cultural differences in health.* Routledge: London.

Kershaw, T. S., Mood, D. W., Newth, G., Ronis, D. L., Sanda, M. G., Vaishampayan, U., & Northouse, L. L. (2008). Longitudinal analysis of a model to predict quality of life in prostate cancer patients and their spouses. *Annals of Behavioral Medicine, 36*(2), 117–128. doi:10.1007/s12160-008-9058-3

Kleiboer, A. M., Kuijer, R. G., Hox, J. J., Schreurs, K. M. G., & Bensing, J. M. (2006). Receiving and providing support in couples dealing with multiple sclerosis: A diary study using an equity perspective. *Personal Relationships, 13*(4), 485–501. doi:10.1111/j.1475-6811.2006.00131.x

Kiecolt-Glaser, J. K., Dura, J. R., Speicher, C. E., Trask, O. J., & Glaser, R. (1991). Spousal caregivers of dementia victims: Longitudinal changes in immunity and health. *Psychosomatic Medicine, 53*(4), 345–362.

Kiecolt-Glaser, J. K., & Newton, T. (2001). Marriage and health: His and hers. *Psychological Bulletin, 127,* 472–503. doi:10.1037/0033-2909.127.4.472

Kim, Y., Carver, C. S., & Cannady, R. S. (2015). Caregiving motivation predicts long-term spirituality and quality of life of the caregivers. *Annals of Behavioral Medicine, 121*(2), 1–10. doi:10.1007/s12160-014-9674-z

Kim, Y., Carver, C. S., Deci, E. L., & Kasser, T. (2008). Adult attachment and psychological well-being in cancer caregivers: The mediational role of spouses' motives for caregiving. *Health Psychology, 27,* 144–154. doi:10.1037/0278-6133.27.2(Suppl.).S144

Kim, Y., Carver, C. S., Rocha-Lima, C., & Shaffer, K. M. (2013). Depressive symptoms among caregivers of colorectal cancer patients during the first year since diagnosis: A longitudinal investigation. *Psycho-Oncology, 22*(2), 362–367. doi:10.1002/pon.2100

Kim, Y., Carver, C. S., Shaffer, K. M., Gansler, T., & Cannady, R. S. (2015b). Cancer caregiving predicts physical impairments: Roles of earlier caregiving stress and being a spousal caregiver. *Cancer, 121*(2), 302–310. doi:10.1002/cncr.29040

Kim, Y., Duberstein, P. R., Sörensen, S., & Larson, M. R. (2005). Levels of depressive symptoms in spouses of people with lung cancer: Effects of personality, social support, and caregiving burden. *Psychosomatics, 46*, 123–130. doi:10.1176/appi.psy.46.2.123

Kim, Y., Kashy, D. A., & Evans, T. V. (2007). Age and attachment style impact stress and depressive symptoms among caregivers: A prospective investigation. *Journal of Cancer Survivorship: Research and Practice, 1*, 35–43. doi10.1007/s11764-007-0011-4

Kim, Y., Loscalzo, M. J., Wellisch, D. K., & Spillers, R. L. (2006). Gender differences in caregiving stress among caregivers of cancer survivors. *Psycho-Oncology, 15*(12), 1086–1092. doi:10.1002/pon.1049

Kim Y., Pavlish, C., Evangelista, L. S., Kopple, J. D., & Phillips, L. R. (2012). Racial/ethnic differences in illness perceptions in minority patients undergoing maintenance hemodialysis. *Nephrology Nursing Journal, 39*(1), 39–49.

Kim, Y., Shaffer, K. M., Carver, C. S., & Cannady, R. S. (2014). Prevalence and predictors of depressive symptoms among cancer caregivers 5 years after the relative's cancer diagnosis. *Journal of Consulting & Clinical Psychology, 82*(1), 1–8. doi:10.1037/a0035116

Kim, Y., Shaffer, K. M., Carver, C. S., & Cannady, R. S. (2015). Quality of life of family caregivers 8 years after a relative's cancer diagnosis: Follow-up of the National Quality of Life Survey for Caregivers. *Psycho-Oncology.* doi:10.1002/pon.3843

Kim, Y., van Ryn, M., Jensen, R. E., Griffin, J. M., Potosky, A. & Rowland, J. (2015a). Effects of gender and depressive symptoms on quality of life among colorectal and lung cancer patients and their family caregivers. *Psycho-Oncology, 24*, 95–105. doi:10.1002/pon.3580

Kneebone, I. I., & Martin, P. R. (2003). Coping and caregivers of people with dementia. *British Journal of Health Psychology, 8*(1), 1–17. doi:10.1348/135910703762879174

Knight, B. G., & Sayegh, P. (2010). Cultural values and caregiving: The updated sociocultural stress and coping model. *The Journals of Gerontology Series B: Psychological Sciences and Social Sciences, 65*(1), 5–13. doi:10.1093/geronb/gbp096

Kobasa, S. C., Maddi, S. R., & Kahn, S. (1982). Hardiness and health: A prospective study. *Journal of Personality & Social Psychology, 42*, 168–177. doi:10.1037/0022-3514.42.1.168

Koerner, S. S., Kenyon, D. B., & Shirai, Y. (2009). Caregiving for elder relatives: Which caregivers experience personal benefits/gains?

Archives of Gerontology and Geriatrics, 48, 238–245. doi:10.1016/j.archger.2008.01.015

Koerner, S. S., & Shirai, Y. (2012). The negative impact of global perceptions of and daily care related family conflict on Hispanic caregivers: Familism as a potential moderator. *Aging & Mental Health, 16*(4), 486–499. doi:10.1080/13607863.2011.638905

Kuijer, R., Buunk, B., & Ybema, J. (2001). Are equity concerns important in the intimate relationship when one partner of a couple has cancer? *Social Psychology Quarterly, 64*(3), 267–282. doi:10.2307/3090116

Kuijer, R. G., Ybema, J. F., Buunk, B. P., De Jong, G. M., Thijs-Boer, F., & Sanderman, R. (2000). Active engagement, protective buffering, and overprotection: Three ways of giving support by intimate partners of patients with cancer. *Journal of Social and Clinical Psychology, 19*(2), 256–275. doi:10.1521/jscp.2000.19.2.256

Kunce, L., & Shaver, P. R. (1994). An attachment-theoretical approach to caregiving in romantic relationships. In K. Bartholomew & D. Perlman (Eds.), *Attachment processes in adulthood: Advances in personal relationships* (pp. 205–237). London: Jessica Kingsley Publishers.

Kuo, B. C. H. (2013). Collectivism and coping: Current theories, evidence, and measurements of collective coping. *International Journal of Psychology, 48*(3), 374–388. doi:10.1080/00207594.2011.640681

Lai, D. W. L. (2010). Filial piety, caregiving appraisal, and caregiving burden. *Research on Aging, 32*(2), 200–223. doi:10.1177/0164027509351475

Lakey, B. (2013). Social support processes in relationships. In J. Simpson & L. Campbell (Eds.), *The Oxford handbook of close relationships* (pp. 710–728). Oxford: Oxford University Press. doi:10.1093/oxfordhb/9780195398694.001.0001

Langer, S. L., Brown, J. D., & Syrjala, K. L. (2009). Intrapersonal and interpersonal consequences of protective buffering among cancer patients and caregivers. *Cancer, 115*(18), 4311–4325. doi:10.1002/cncr.24586

Laudenslager, M. L. (2014). "Anatomy of an Illness": Control from a caregiver's perspective. *Brain, Behavior, & Immunity, 36*, 1–8. doi:10.1016/j.bbi.2013.08.012

Laudenslager, M. L., Simoneau, T. L., Kilbourn, K., Natvig, C., Philips, S., Spradley, J., Benitez, P., McSweeney, P., & Mikulich-Gilbertson, S. K. (2015). A randomized control trial of a psychosocial intervention for caregivers of allogeneic hematopoietic stem cell transplant patients: Effects on distress. *Bone Marrow Transplantation*, 50, 1110–1118. doi:10.1038/bmt.2015

Laurenceau, J., Barrett, L., & Pietromonaco, P. (1998). Intimacy as an interpersonal process: The importance of self-disclosure, partner disclosure, and perceived partner responsiveness in interpersonal exchanges. *Journal of Personality & Social Psychology, 74*(5), 1238–1251. doi:10.1037/0022-3514.74.5.1238

Lawang, W., Horey, D. E., & Blackford, J. (2015). Family caregivers of adults with acquired physical disability: Thai case-control study. *International Journal of Nursing Practice, 21*(1), 70–77. doi:10.1111/ijn.12215

Lawang, W., Horey, D., Blackford, J., Sunsern, R., & Riewpaiboon, W. (2013). Support interventions for caregivers of physically disabled adults: A systematic review. *Nursing & Health Sciences, 15*, 534–545. doi:10.1111/nhs.12063

Lawrence, J. A., Goodnow, J. J., Woods, K., & Karantzas, G. (2002). Distributions of caregiving tasks among family members: The place of gender and availability. *Journal of Family Psychology, 16*(4), 493–509. doi:10.1037/0893-3200.16.4.493

Lawton, M. P., Moss, M., Hoffman, C., & Perkinson, M. (2000). Two transitions in daughters' caregiving careers. *The Gerontologist, 40*(4), 437–448. doi:10.1093/geront/40.4.437.

Lazarus, R. S., & Folkman, S. (1984). *Stress, appraisal, and coping.* New York: Springer.

Lee, C. S., Vellone, E., Lyons, K. S., Cocchieri, A., Bidwell, J. T., D'Agostino, F., Hiatt, S. O., Alvaro, R., Buck, H. G., & Riegel, B. (2015). Patterns and predictors of patient and caregiver engagement in heart failure care: A multi-level dyadic study. *International Journal of Nursing Studies, 52*, 588–597. doi:10.1016/j.ijnurstu.2014.11.005

Legg, L. A., Quinn, T. J., Mahmood, F., Weir, C. J., Tierney, J., Stott, D. J., Smith, L. N., & Langhorne, P. (2011). Non-pharmacological interventions for caregivers of stroke survivors. *Cochrane Database of Systematic Reviews, 10*. doi:10.1002/14651858.CD008179.pub2

Lethborg, C. E., Kissane, D., & Burns, W. I. (2003). "It's Not the Easy Part": The experience of significant others of women with early stage breast cancer, at treatment completion. *Social Work in Health Care, 37*(1), 63–85. doi:10.1300/J010v37n01_04

Lepore, S. (2001). A social-cognitive processing model of emotional adjustment to cancer. In A. Baum & B. Andersen (Eds.), *Psychosocial interventions for cancer* (pp. 99–118). Washington, DC: APA. doi:10.1037/10402-006

Lepore, S. J., & Revenson, T. A. (2006). Resilience and posttraumatic growth: Recovery, resistance, & reconfiguration. In L. Calhoun & R. G. Tedeschi (Eds.), *The handbook of posttraumatic growth: Research and practice* (pp. 24–46). Mahwah, NJ: Erlbaum.

Leventhal, H., Bodnar-Deren, S., Breland, J. Y., Hash-Converse, J., Phillips, L. A., Leventhal, E. A., & Cameron, L. D. (2012). Modeling health and illness behavior: The approach of the Commonsense Model. In A. Baum, T. A. Revenson, & J. E. Singer (Eds.), *Handbook of health psychology*, 2nd edition (pp. 3–35). New York: Psychology Press.

Li, J., Ngin, P. M., & Teo, A. C. (2008). Culture and leadership in Singapore: Combination of the East and the West. In J. S. Chokar., F. C. Brodbeck & R. J. House (Eds.), *Culture and leadership across the world: The GLOBE book of in-depth studies of 25 countries* (pp. 947–968). Mahway, NJ: Lawrence Erlbaum.

Li, L. W. (2005). From caregiving to bereavement: Trajectories of depressive symptoms among wife and daughter caregivers. *The Journals of Gerontology Series B: Psychological Sciences and Social Sciences, 60*(4), 190–198. doi:10.1093/geronb/60.4.P190

Li, Q. & Loke, A. Y. (2013a). A spectrum of hidden morbidities among spousal caregivers for patients with cancer, and differences between the genders: A review of the literature. *European Journal of Oncology Nursing, 17*(5), 578–587. doi:10.1016/j.ejon.2013.01.007

Li, Q. & Loke, A. Y. (2013b). The positive aspects of caregiving for cancer patients: A critical review of the literature and directions for future research. *Psycho-Oncology, 22*(11), 2399–2407. doi:10.1002/pon.3311

Li, Q. P., Mak, Y. W., & Loke, A. Y. (2013). Spouses' experience of caregiving for cancer patients: A literature review. *International Nursing Review, 60*(2), 178–187. doi:10.1111/inr.12000

Libert, Y., Merckaert, I., Slachmuylder, J., & Razavi, D. (2013). The ability of informal primary caregivers to accurately report cancer patients' difficulties. *Psycho-Oncology, 22*(12), 2840–2847. doi:10.1002/pon.3362

Lin, I. F., Fee, H. R., & Wu, H. S. (2012). Negative and positive caregiving experiences: A closer look at the intersection of gender and relationship. *Family Relations, 61*(2), 343–358. doi:10.1111/j.1741-3729.2011.00692.x

Lindstrom, K. B., & Mazurek-Melnyk, B. (2013). Feasibility and preliminary effects of an intervention targeting schema development for caregivers of newly admitted hospice patients. *Journal of Palliative Medicine, 16,* 680–685. doi:10.1089/jpm.2012.0198

Liu, J., Guo, M., & Bern-Klug, M. (2013). Economic stress among adult-child caregivers of the oldest old in China: The importance of contextual factors. *Journal of Cross-cultural Gerontology, 28*(4), 465–479. doi:10.1007/s10823-013-9216-3

Liu, Y., Insel, K. S., Reed, P. G., & Crist, J. D. (2012). Family caregiving of older people. Chinese people with dementia: Testing a model. *Nursing Research, 61*(1), 39–50. doi:10.1097/NNR.0b013e31823bc451

Lockenhoff, C. E., Duberstein, P. R., Friedman, B., & Costa, P. T. (2011). Five-factor personality traits and subjective health among caregivers: The role of caregiver strain and self-efficacy. *Psychology & Aging, 26,* 592–604. doi:10.1037/a0022209

Lopez, V., Copp, G., & Molassiotis, A. (2012). Male caregivers of patients with breast and gynecologic cancer: Experiences from caring for their spouses and partners. *Cancer Nursing, 35*(6), 402–410. doi:10.1097/NCC.0b013e318231daf0

Lopez-Hartmann, M., Wens, J., Verhoeven, V., & Remmen, R. (2012). The effect of caregiver support interventions for informal caregivers of community-dwelling frail elderly: A systematic review. *International Journal of Integrated Care, 12,* 1–16.

Lord, K., Livingston, G., & Cooper, C. (2015). A systematic review of barriers and facilitators to and interventions for proxy decision-making by family carers of people with dementia. *International Psychogeriatrics, 27*(8), 1301–1312. doi:10.1017/S1041610215000411

Lutgendorf, S. K., & Laudenslager, M. L. (2009). Care of the caregiver: Stress and dysregulation of inflammatory control in cancer caregivers. *Journal of Clinical Oncology, 27*(18), 2894–2895. doi:10.1200/JCO.2009.22.1523

Lyonette, C., & Yardley, L. (2003). The influence on carer wellbeing of motivations to care for older people and the relationship. *Ageing & Society, 23*(4), 487–506. doi:10.1017/S0144686X03001284

Lyons, J. G., Cauley, J. A., & Fredman, L. (2015). The effect of transitions in caregiving status and intensity on perceived stress among 992 female caregivers and noncaregivers. *The Journals of Gerontology Series A: Biological Sciences and Medical Sciences, 70*(8). doi:10.1093/gerona/glv001

Lyons, K., Zarit, S., Sayer, A., & Whitlatch, C. (2002). Caregiving as a dyadic process: Perspectives from caregiver and receiver. *The Journals* of Gerontology Series B:-Psychological Sciences and Social Sciences, 57(3), 195–204. doi:10.1093/geronb/57.3.P195

Macintyre, S., & Hunt, K. (1997). Socio-economic position, gender and health how do they interact? *Journal of Health Psychology, 2*(3), 315–334. doi:10.1177/135910539700200304

Mackenzie, A., & Greenwood, N. (2012). Positive experiences of caregiving in stroke: A systematic review. *Disability & Rehabilitation, 34*(17), 1413–1422. doi:10.3109/09638288.2011.650307

MacNeil, G., Kosberg, J. I., Durkin, D. W., Dooley, W. K., DeCoster, J., & Williamson, G. M. (2010). Caregiver mental health and potentially harmful caregiving behavior: The central role of caregiver anger. *The Gerontologist, 50*(1), 76–86. doi:10.1093/geront/gnp099

Magai, C., & Cohen, C. I. (1998). Attachment style and emotion regulation in dementia patients and their relation to caregiver burden. *The Journals of Gerontology Series B: Psychological Sciences and Social Sciences of Gerontology, 53*, 147–154. doi:10.1093/geronb/53B.3.P147

Malhotra, R., Chan, A., Malhotra, C., & Østbye, T. (2012). Validity and reliability of the Caregiver Reaction Assessment scale among primary informal caregivers for older persons in Singapore. *Aging & Mental Health, 16*(8), 1004–1015. doi:10.1080/13607863.2012.702728

Mallinger, J. B., Griggs, J. J., & Shields, C. G. (2006). Family communication and mental health after breast cancer. *European Journal of Cancer Care, 15*(4), 355–361. doi:10.1111/j.1365-2354.2006.00666.x

Manne, S., & Badr, H. (2008). Intimacy and relationship processes in couples' psychosocial adaptation to cancer. *Cancer, 112*(11), 2541–2555. doi:10.1002/cncr.23450

Manne, S., Badr, H., & Kashy, D. A. (2012). A longitudinal analysis of intimacy processes and psychological distress among couples coping with head and neck or lung cancers. *Journal of Behavioral Medicine, 35*(3), 334–346. doi:10.1007/s10865-011-9349-1

Manne, S., Badr, H., Zaider, T., Nelson, C., & Kissane, D. (2010). Cancer-related communication, relationship intimacy, and psychological distress among couples coping with localized prostate cancer. *Journal of Cancer Survivorship-Research and Practice, 4*(1), 74–85. doi:10.1007/s11764-009-0109-y

Manne, S. L., Norton, T. R., Winkel, G., Ostroff, J. S., Fox, K., & Grana, G. (2007). Protectective buffering and psychological distress among couples coping with breast cancer: The moderating role of relationship satisfaction. *Journal of Family Psychology, 21*(3), 380–388. doi:10.1037/0893-3200.21.3.380

Manne, S., Ostroff, J., Rini, C., Fox, K., Goldstein, L., & Grana, G. (2004). The interpersonal process model of intimacy: The role of self-disclosure, partner disclosure, and partner responsiveness in interactions between breast cancer patients and their partners. *Journal of Family Psychology, 18*(4), 589–599. doi:10.1037/0893-3200.18.4.589

Manne, S., Ostroff, J., Norton, T., Fox, K., Goldstein, L., & Grana, G. (2006). Cancer-related relationship communication in couples coping with early stage breast cancer. *Psycho-Oncology, 15*(3), 234–247. doi:10.1002/pon.941

Manne, S., Ostroff, J., Sherman, M., Heyman, R., Ross, S., & Fox, K. (2004). Couples' support-related communication, psychological distress, and relationship satisfaction among women with early stage breast cancer. *Journal of Consulting and Clinical Psychology, 72*(4), 660–670. doi:10.1037/0022-006X.72.4.660

Manne, S. L., Siegel, S., Kashy, D., & Heckman, C. J. (2014). Cancer-specific relationship awareness, relationship communication, and intimacy among couples coping with early-stage breast cancer. *Journal of Social and Personal Relationships, 31*(3), 314–334. doi:10.1177/0265407513494950

Martín-Martín, L. M., Valenza-Demet, G., Ariza-Vega, P., Valenza, C., Castellote-Caballero, Y., & Jiménez-Moleó, J. J. (2014). Effectiveness of an occupational therapy intervention in reducing emotional distress in informal caregivers of hip fracture patients: A randomized controlled trial. *Clinical Rehabilitation, 28*, 772–783. doi:10.1177/0269215513519343

Martire, L. M., Schulz, R., Helgeson, V. S., Small, B. J., & Saghafi, E. (2010). Review and meta-analysis of couple-oriented interventions for chronic illness. *Annals of Behavioral Medicine, 40*, 325–342. doi:10.1007/s12160-010-9216-2.

Mason, A., Weatherly, H., Spilsbury, K., Golder, S., Arksey, H., Adamson, J., & Drummond, M. (2007). The effectiveness and cost-effectiveness of respite for caregivers of frail older people. *Journal of American Geriatric Society, 55*, 290–299. doi:10.1111/j.1532-5415.2006.01037.

Maunder, R. G., & Hunter, J. J. (2001). Attachment and psychosomatic medicine: Developmental contributions to stress and disease. *Psychosomatic Medicine, 63*, 556–567. doi:10.1097/00006842-200107000-00006

Maunder, R. G., & Hunter, J. J. (2008). Attachment relationships as determinants of physical health. *The Journal of the American Academy of Psychoanalysis and Dynamic Psychiatry, 36,* 11–32. doi:10.1521/jaap.2008.36.1.11

Mausbach, B. T., von Konel, R., Roepke, S. K., Moore, R., Patterson, T. L., Mills, P. J., Dimsdale, J. E., Ziegler, M. G., Ancoli-Israel, S., Allison, M., & Grant, I. (2011). Self-efficacy buffers the relationship between dementia caregiving stress and circulating concentrations of the proinflammatory cytokine interleukin-6. *American Journal of Geriatric Psychiatry, 19,* 64–71. doi:10.1097/JGP.0b013e3181df4498

McClendon, M. J., & Smyth, K. A. (2013). Quality of informal care for persons with dementia: Dimensions and correlates. *Aging & Mental Health, 17,* 1003–1015. doi:10.1080/13607863.2013.805400

McCrae, R. R., & Costa, P. T. (2003). *Personality in adulthood: A five-factor theory perspective.* New York: Guilford Press.

McMillan, S. C., Small, B. J., Weitzner, M., Schonwetter, R., Tittle, M., Moody, L., & Haley, W. E. (2006). Impact of coping skills intervention with family caregivers of hospice patients with cancer. A randomized clinical trial. *Cancer, 106*(1), 214–222. doi:10.1002/cncr.21567

Melo, G., Maroco, J., & De Mendoza, A. (2011). Influence of personality on caregiver's burden, depression and distress related to the BPSD. *Journal of Geriatric Psychiatry, 26,* 1275–1282. doi:10.1002/gps.2677

Menne, H. L., & Whitlatch, C. J. (2007). Decision-making involvement of individuals with dementia. *Gerontologist, 47*(6), 810–819. doi:10.1093/geront/47.6.810

Mestheneos, E., Triantafillou, J., and the EUROFAMCARE group (2005). Supporting Family Carers of Older People in Europe – the Pan-European Background. http://www.uke.de/extern/eurofamcare/documents/nabares/peubare_a4.pdf. Retrieved June 28, 2015.

MetLife Mature Market Institute, National Alliance for Caregiving, & The National Center on Women and Aging. (1999). The Metlife juggling act study: Balancing caregiving with work and the costs involved. Cited in Family Caregiver Alliance (2015). Women and Caregiving: Facts and Figures. https://caregiver.org/women-and-caregiving-facts-and-figures. Retrieved July 2, 2015.

Michela, J. L. (1987). Interpersonal and individual and impacts of a husband's heart attack. In A. Baum & J. E. Singer (Eds.), *Handbook of psychology and health,* vol. 5 (pp. 255–301). Mahwah, NJ: Erlbaum.

Mikulincer, M., Ein-Dor, T., Solomon, Z., & Shaver, P. R. (2011). Trajectories of attachment insecurities over a 17-year period: A latent growth curve Analysis of the Impact of war captivity and posttraumatic stress disorder. *Journal of Social and Clinical Psychology, 30*, 960–984. doi:10.1521/jscp.2011.30.9.960

Mikulincer, M., & Shaver, P. R. (2007). *Attachment patterns in adulthood: Structure, dynamics, and change.* New York: Guilford Press.

Mikulincer, M., & Shaver, P. R. (2009). An attachment and behavioral systems perspective on social support. *Journal of Social and Personal Relationships, 26*, 7–19. doi:10.1177/0265407509105518

Mikulincer, M., Shaver, P. R., Gillath, O., & Nitzberg, R. (2005). Attachment, caregiving, and altruism: Boosting attachment security increases compassion and helping. *Journal of Personality & Social Psychology, 89*, 817–839. doi:10.1037/0022-3514.89.5.817

Miller, B., & Cafasso, L. (1992). Gender differences in caregiving: Fact or artifact? *The Gerontologist, 32*, 498–507. doi:10.1093/geront/32.4.498

Mitchell, M. M., Robinson, A. C., Wolff, J. L., & Knowlton, A. R. (2014). Perceived mental health status of drug users with HIV: Concordance between caregivers and care recipient reports and associations with caregiving burden and reciprocity. *Aids & Behavior, 18*(6), 1103–1113. doi:10.1007/s10461-013-0681-z

Mittleman, M. (2005). Taking care of the caregivers. *Current Opinions in Psychiatry, 18*, 633–639. doi:10.1097/01.yco.0000184416.21458.40

Moen, P., Robison, J., & Dempster-McClain, D. (1995). Caregiving and women's well-being: A life course approach. *Journal of Health & Social Behavior, 36*(3), 259–273. doi:10.2307/2137342

Monahan, D. J., & Hooker, K. (1995). Health of spouse caregivers of dementia patients: The role of personality and social support. *Social Work, 40*, 305–314. doi: 10.1093/sw/40.3.305

Monin, J. K., Martire, L. M., Schulz, R., & Clark, M. S. (2009). Willingness to express emotions to caregiving spouses. *Emotion 9*(1), 101–106. doi:10.1037/a0013732

Monin, J. K., Schulz, R., & Kershaw, T. S. (2013). Caregiving spouses' attachment orientations and the physical and psychological health of individuals with Alzheimer's disease. *Aging & Mental Health, 17*, 508–516. doi:10.1080/13607863.2012.747080

Monroe, S. M., & Simons, A. D. (1991). Diathesis-stress theories in the context of life stress research: Implications for the depressive disorders. *Psychological Bulletin, 110*, 406–425. doi:10.1037/0033-2909.110.3.406

Moon, H., & Adams, K. B. (2013). The effectiveness of dyadic interventions for people with dementia and their caregivers. *Dementia-International Journal of Social Research and Practice, 12*(6), 821–839. doi:10.1177/1471301212447026

Morse, J. Q., Shaffer, D. R., Williamson, G. M., Dooley, W. K., & Schulz, R. (2012(. Models of self and others and their relation to positive and negative caregiving responses. *Psychology & Aging, 27,* 211–218. doi:10.1037/a0023960

Morrison, V., Ager, A., & Willock, J. (1999). Perceived risk of tropical disease in Malawi: Evidence of unrealistic pessimism and the irrelevance of beliefs of personal control. *Psychology, Health & Medicine, 4*(4), 361–368. doi:10.1080/135485099106108

Morrison, V., & Bennett P. (2012). *Introduction to health psychology*, 3rd edition. Harlow, England: Pearson Education Limited.

Moser, M. T., Künzler, A., Nussbeck, F., Bargetzi, M., & Znoj, H. J. (2013). Higher emotional distress in female partners of cancer patients: Prevalence and patient–partner interdependencies in a 3-year cohort. *Psycho-Oncology, 22*(12), 2693–2701. doi:10.1002/pon.3331

Mui, A. C. (1995). Caring for frail elderly parents: A comparison of adult sons and daughters. *The Gerontologist, 35*(1), 86–93. doi:10.1093/geront/35.1.86

Nagpal, N., Heid, A. R., Zarit, S. H., & Whitlatch, C. J. (2015). Religiosity and quality of life: A dyadic perspective of individuals with dementia and their caregivers. *Aging & Mental Health, 19,* 500–506. doi:10.1080/13607863.2014.952708

National Alliance for Caregiving and AARP. (2015). Caregiving in the U.S. 2015. Bethesda, MD: National Alliance for Caregiving.

National Alliance for Caregiving, University of Pittsburgh Institute on Aging, & the MetLife Mature Market Institute (2010). The MetLife Study of Working Caregivers and Employer Health Care Costs. NY: Metlife Mature Market Institute. https://www.metlife.com/assets/cao/mmi/publications/studies/2010/mmi-working-caregivers-employers-health-care-costs.pdf. Retrieved July 2, 2015

Neugaard, B., Andresen, E., McKune, S. L., & Jamoom, E. W. (2008). Health-related quality of life in a national sample of caregivers: Findings from the behavioral risk factor surveillance system. *Journal of Happiness Studies, 9*(4), 559–575. doi:10.1007/s10902-008-9089-2

Neugarten, B. (1979). Time, age and the life cycle. *American Journal of Psychiatry, 136,* 887–894. doi:10.1176/ajp.136.7.887

Nelis, S. M., Clare, L., & Whitaker, C. J. (2012). Attachment representations in people with dementia and their carers: Implications for well-being within the dyad. *Aging & Mental Health, 16*, 845–854. doi:10.1080/13607863.2012.667779

New York State Office for the Aging. (2012). Caregiver training resources. http://www.nyscrc.org/documents/CaregiverTrainingResourcesProject.pdf. Retrieved June 26, 2015

Nijboer, C., Tempelaar, R., Triemstra, M., van den Bos, G. A., & Sanderman, R. (2001). The role of social and psychologic resources in caregiving of cancer patients. *Cancer, 91*(5), 1029–1039. doi:10.1002/1097-0142(20010301)91:5<1029::AID-CNCR1094>3.0.CO;2-1

Nolen-Hoeksema, S. (2001). Gender differences in depression. *Current Directions in Psychological Science, 10*(5), 173–176. doi:10.1111/1467-8721.00142

Northouse, L. L., Katapodi, M. C., Song, L., Zhang, L., & Mood, D. W. (2010). Interventions with caregivers of cancer patients: Meta-analysis of randomized trials. *CA: A Cancer Journal for Clinicians, 60*, 317–339. doi:10.3322/caac.20081

Northouse, L., Williams, A. L., Given, B., & McCorkle, R. (2012). Psychosocial care for family caregivers of patients with cancer. *Journal of Clinical Oncology, 30*(11), 1227–1234. doi:10.1200/JCO.2011.39.5798

O'Dwyer, S. T., Moyle, W., Zimmer-Gembeck, M., & De Leo, D. (2013). Suicidal ideation in family carers of people with dementia: A pilot study. *International Journal of Geriatric Psychiatry, 28*, 1182–1188. doi:10.1002/gps.3941

Orbach, D. (2007) Committed to caring: older women and HIV and AIDS in Cambodia, Thailand and Vietnam. London: HelpAge International. http://www.helpage.org/Researchandpolicy/HIVAIDS/Resources. Retrieved July 15, 2015.

Orgeta, V., & Leung, P. (2015). Personality and dementia caring. *Current Opinion in Psychiatry, 28*, 57–65. doi:10.1097/YCO.0000000000000116

Ouellette, S. C., & DiPlacido, J. (2001). Personality's role in the protection and enhancement of health: Where the research has been, where it is stuck, how it might move. In A. Baum, T. A. Revenson, & J. Singer (Eds.), *Handbook of health psychology* (pp. 175–193). Mahwah, NJ: Erlbaum.

Pailler, M. E., Johnson, T. M., Zevon, M. A., Kuszczak, S., Griffiths, E., Thompson, J., Wang, E. S., & Wetzler, M. (2015). Acceptability, feasibility and efficacy of a supportive group intervention for caregivers of newly diagnosed leukemia patients. *Journal of Psychosocial Oncology, 33*, 163–177. doi:10.1080/07347332.2014.99208

Papastavrou, E., Charalambous, A., & Tsangari, H. (2012). How do informal caregivers of patients with cancer cope: A descriptive study of the coping strategies employed. *European Journal of Oncology Nursing, 16*(3), 258–263. doi:10.1016/j.ejon.2011.06.001

Parveen, S., & Morrison, V. (2009). Predictors of familism: A pilot study. *Journal of Health Psychology, 14*(8), 1135–1143. doi:10.1177/1359105309343020

Parveen, S., & Morrison, V. (2012). Predicting caregiver gains: A longitudinal study. *British Journal of Health Psychology, 17*(4), 711–723. doi:10.1111/j.2044-8287.2012.02067.x

Parveen, S., Morrison, V., & Robinson, C. A. (2011). Ethnic variations in the caregiver role: A qualitative study. *Journal of Health Psychology, 16*(6), 862–872. doi:10.1177/1359105310392416

Parveen, S., Morrison, V., & Robinson, C. A. (2013). Ethnicity, familism and willingness to care: Important influences on caregiver mood? *Aging & Mental Health, 17*(1), 115–124. doi:10.1080/13607863.2012.717251

Parveen, S., Morrison, V., & Robinson, C. A. (2014). Does coping mediate the relationship between familism and caregiver outcomes. *Aging & Mental Health, 18*(2), 255–259. doi:10.1080/13607863.2013.827626

Pasipanodya, E. C., Parrish, B. P., Laurenceau, J., Cohen, L. H., Siegel, S. D., Graber, E. C., & Belcher, A. J. (2012). Social constraints on disclosure predict daily well-being in couples coping with early-stage breast cancer. *Journal of Family Psychology, 26*(4), 661–667. doi:10.1037/a0028655

Patrick, J., & Hayden, J. (1999). Neuroticism, coping strategies, and negative well-being among caregivers. *Psychology & Aging, 14*, 273–283. doi:10.1037/0882-7974.14.2.273

Pearlin, L. I. (1989). Sociological study of stress. *Journal of Health and Social Behavior, 30*, 241–256. doi:10.2307/2136956

Pearlin, L. I., & Skaff, M. M. (1995). *Stressors and adaptation in late life.* Washington, DC: APA

Pearlin, L. I., Mullan, J. T., Semple, S. J., & Skaff, M. M. (1990). Caregiving and the stress process: An overview of concepts and their measures. *The Gerontologist, 30*(5), 583–594. doi:10.1093/geront/30.5.583

Penner, L. A., Cline, R. J. W., Albrecht, T. L., Harper, F. W. K., Peterson, A. M., Taub, J. M., & Ruckdeschel, J. C. (2008). Parents' empathic responses and pain and distress in pediatric patients. *Basic & Applied Social Psychology, 30*(2), 102–113. doi:10.1080/01973530802208824

Perren, S., Schmid, R., Herrmann, S., & Wettstein, A. (2007). The impact of attachment on dementia-related problem behavior and spousal caregivers' well-being. *Attachment & Human Development, 9*, 163–178. doi:10.1080/14616730701349630

Piccinelli, M., & Wilkinson, G. (2000). Gender differences in depression: Critical review. *The British Journal of Psychiatry, 177*(6), 486–492. doi:10.1192/bjp.177.6.486

Piercy, K. W., Fauth, E. B., Norton, M. C., Pfister, R., Corcoran, C. D., Rabins, P. V., Lyketsos, C., & Tschanz, J. T. (2013). Predictors of dementia caregiver depressive symptoms in a population: The Cache County Dementia Progression Study. *The Journals of Gerontology Series B: Psychological Sciences and Social Sciences, 68*(6), 921–926. doi:10.1093/geronb/gbs116

Pietromonaco, P. R., Uchino, B., & Dunkel Schetter, C. (2013). Close relationship processes and health: Implications of attachment theory for health and disease. *Health Psychology, 32*, 499–513. doi:10.1037/a0029349

Pihl, E., Jacobsson, A., Fridlund, B., Strömberg, A., & Måtensson, J. (2005). Depression and health-related quality of life in elderly patients suffering from heart failure and their spouses: A comparative study. *European Journal of Heart Failure, 7*(4), 583–589. doi:10.1016/j.ejheart.2004.07.016

Piil, K., Juhler, M., Jakobsen, J., & Jarden, M. (2014). Controlled rehabilitative and supportive care intervention trials in patients with high-grade gliomas and their caregivers: A systematic review. *BMJ Supportive & Palliative Care. Advance online publication*. doi:10.1136/bmjspcare-2013-000593

Pinquart, M., & Sörensen, S. (2003). Associations of stressors and uplifts of caregiving with caregiver burden and depressive mood: A meta-analysis. *The Journals of Gerontology Series B: Psychological Sciences and Social Sciences, 58*(2), 112–128. doi:10.1093/geronb/58.2.P112

Pinquart, M., & Sörensen, S. (2005). Ethnic differences in stressors, resources, and psychological outcomes of family caregiving: A meta-analysis. *The Gerontologist, 45*(1), 90–106. doi:10.1093/geront/45.1.90

Pinquart, M., & Sörensen S. (2006). Gender differences in caregiver stressors, social resources, and health: An updated meta-analysis. *The Journals of Gerontology, Series B: Psychological Sciences and Social Sciences, 61*, 33–45. doi:10.1093/geronb/61.1.P33

Pinquart, M., & Sörensen, S. (2007). Correlates of physical health of informal caregivers: A meta-analysis. *The Journals of Gerontology Series B: Psychological Sciences and Social Sciences, 62*(2), 126–137. doi:10.1093/geronb/62.2.P126

Pinquart, M., & Sörensen, S. (2011). Spouses, adult children, and children-in-law as caregivers of older adults: A meta-analytic comparison. *Psychology & Aging, 26*(1), 1–14. doi:10.1037/a0021863

Pirraglia, P. A., Bishop, D., Herman, D. S., Trisvan, E., Lopez, R. A., Torgersen, C. S., Van Hof, A. M., Anderson, B. J., Miller, I., & Stein, M. D. (2005). Caregiver burden and depression among informal caregivers of HIV-infected individuals. *Journal of General Internal Medicine, 20*(6), 510–514. doi:10.1111/j.1525-1497.2005.0073.x

Porter, L. S., Keefe, F. J., Baucom, D. H., Hurwitz, H., Moser, B., Patterson, E., & Kim, H. J. (2009). Partner-assisted emotional disclosure for patients with gastrointestinal cancer results from a randomized controlled trial. *Cancer, 115*(18), 4326–4338. doi:10.1002/cncr.24578

Porter, L. S., Keefe, F. J., Davis, D., Rumble, M., Scipio, C., & Garst, J. (2012). Attachment styles in patients with lung cancer and their spouses: Associations with patient and spouse adjustment. *Supportive Care in Cancer, 20*, 2459–2466 . doi:10.1007/s00520-011-1367-6

Porter, L. S., Keefe, F. J., Hurwitz, H., & Faber, M. (2005). Disclosure between patients with gastrointestinal cancer and their spouses. *Psycho-Oncology, 14*(12), 1030–1042. doi:10.1002/pon.915

Pottie, C. G., Burch, K. A., Montross Thomas, L. P., & Irwin, S. A. (2014). Informal caregiving of hospice patients. *Journal of Palliative Medicine, 17*(7), 845–856. doi:10.1089/jpm.2013.0196

Pressler, S. J., Gradus-Pizlo, I., Chubinski, S. D., Smith, G., Wheeler, S., Wu, J., & Sloan, R. (2009). Family caregiver outcomes in heart failure. *American Journal of Critical Care, 18*(2), 149–159. doi:10.4037/ajcc2009300

Quah, S. H., & Bishop, G. D. (1996). Seeking help for illness the roles of cultural orientation and illness cognition. *Journal of Health Psychology, 1*(2), 209–222. doi.org/10.1177/135910539600100205

Quinn, C., Clare, L., & Woods, R. T. (2010). The impact of motivations and meanings on the wellbeing of caregivers of people with dementia: A systematic review. *International Psychogeriatrics, 22*(1), 43–55. doi:10.1017/S1041610209990810

Rae, H. M. (1998). Managing feelings caregiving as emotion work. *Research on Aging, 20*(1), 137–160. doi:10.1177/0164027598201007

Rabinowitz, Y. G., Saenz, E. C., Thompson, L. W., & Gallagher-Thompson, D. (2011). Understanding caregiver health behaviors: Depressive symptoms mediate caregiver self-efficacy and health behavior patterns. *American Journal of Alzheimer's Disease and Other Dementias, 26*, 310–316. doi:10.1177/1533317511410557

Ramos, B. M. (2004). Culture, ethnicity and caregiver stress among Puerto Ricans. *Journal of Applied Gerontology, 23*(4), 469–486. doi:10.1177/0733464804271281

Raschick, M., & Ingersoll-Dayton, B. (2004). The costs and rewards of caregiving among aging spouses and adult children. *Family Relations, 53*(3), 317–325. doi:10.1111/j.0022-2445.2004.0008.x

Raune, D., Kuipers, E., & Bebbington, P. E. (2004). Expressed emotion at first-episode psychosis: Investigating a carer appraisal model. *British Journal of Psychiatry, 184*(4), 321–326. doi:10.1192/bjp.184.4.321

Reamy, A. M., Kim, K., Zarit, S. H., & Whitlatch, C. J. (2011). Understanding discrepancy in perceptions of values: Individuals with mild to moderate dementia and their family caregivers. *The Gerontologist, 51*(4), 473–483. doi:10.1093/geront/gnr010

Reinhardt, J. P., Boerner, K., & Horowitz, A. (2006). Good to have but not to use: Differential impact of perceived and received support on well-being. *Journal of Social and Personal Relationships, 23*, 117–129. doi:10.1177/0265407506060182

Revenson, T. A. (1990). All other things are not equal: An ecological perspective on the relation between personality and disease. In H. S. Friedman (Ed.), *Personality and disease* (pp. 65–94). New York: John Wiley.

Revenson, T. A. (2003). Scenes from a marriage: Examining support, coping, and gender within the context of chronic illness. In J. Suls, & K. Wallston (Eds.), *Social psychological foundations of health and illness* (pp. 530–559). Oxford, England: Blackwell Publishing. doi:10.1002/9780470753552.ch19

Revenson, T. A., Abraído-Lanza, A. F., Majerovitz, S. D., & Jordan, C. (2005). Couples coping with chronic illness: What's gender got to do with it? In T. A. Revenson, K. Kayser, & G. Bodenmann (Eds.),

Couples coping with stress: Emerging perspectives on dyadic coping (pp. 137–156). Washington, DC: APA. doi:10.1037/11031-007

Revenson, T. A., & DeLongis, A. (2011). Couples coping with chronic illness. In S. Folkman (Ed.), *The Oxford handbook of stress, health, and coping* (pp. 101–126). New York: Oxford University Press.

Rhee, Y., Degenholtz, H. B., Lo Sasso, A. T., & Emanuel, L. L. (2009). Estimating the quantity and economic value of family caregiving for community-dwelling older persons in the last year of life. *Journal of the American Geriatrics Society, 57*(9), 1654–1659. doi:10.1111/j.1532-5415.2009.02390

Rhee, Y. S., Yun, Y. H., Park, S., Shin, D. O., Lee, K. M., Yoo, H. J., Kim, J. H., Kim, S. O., Lee, R., Lee, Y. O., & Kim, N. S. (2008). Depression in family caregivers of cancer patients: The feeling of burden as a predictor of depression. *Journal of Clinical Oncology, 26*(36), 5890–5895. doi:10.1200/JCO.2007.15.3957

Richieri, R., Boyer, L., Reine, G., Loundou, A., Auquier, P., Lancon, C., & Simeoni, M. C. (2011). The Schizophrenia Caregiver Quality of Life questionnaire (S-CGQoL): Development and validation of an instrument to measure quality of life of caregivers of individuals with schizophrenia. *Schizophrenia Research, 126*(1), 192–201. doi:10.1016/j.schres.2010.08.037

Robinson, B. C. (1983). Validation of a caregiver strain index. *Journal of Gerontology, 38*(3), 344–348. doi:10.1093/geronj/38.3.344

Roepke, S. K., Mausbach, B. T., von Knel, R., Ancoli-Israel, S., Harmell, A. L., Dimsdale, J. E., Aschbacher, K., Mills, P. J., Patterson, T. L., & Grant, I. (2009). The moderating role of personal mastery on the relationship between caregiving status and multiple dimensions of fatigue. *International Journal of Geriatric Psychiatry, 24*, 1453–1462. doi:10.1002/gps.2286

Rohr, M. K., Wagner, J., & Lang, F. R. (2013). Effects of personality on the transition into caregiving. *Psychology and Aging, 28*, 692–700. doi:10.1037/a0034133

Romero-Moreno, R., Márquez-González, M., Losada, A., & López, J. (2011). Motives for caring: Relationship to stress and coping dimensions. *International Psychogeriatrics, 23*(4), 573–582. doi:10.1017/S1041610210001821

Romito, F., Goldzweig, G., Cormio, C., Hagedoorn, M., & Andersen, B. L. (2013). Informal caregiving for cancer patients. *Cancer, 119*(S11), 2160–2169. doi:10.1002/cncr.28057

Roth, D. L., Fredman, L., & Haley, W. E. (2015). Informal caregiving and its impact on health: A reappraisal from population-based studies. *The Gerontologist*, gnu177. doi:10.1093/geront/gnu177

Rottmann, N., Hansen, D. G., Larsen, P. V., Nicolaisen, A., Flyger, H., Johansen, C., & Hagedoorn, M. (2015). Dyadic coping within couples dealing with breast cancer: A longitudinal, population-based study. *Health Psychology, 34*(5), 486–495. doi:10.1037/hea0000218

Ruiz, J. M., Matthews, K. A., Scheier, M. F., & Schulz, R. (2006). Does who you marry matter for your health? Influence of patients' and spouses' personality on their partners' psychological well-being following coronary artery bypass surgery. *Journal of Personality and Social Psychology, 91*, 255–267. doi:10.1037/0022-3514.91.2.255

Ryan, R. M., & Deci, E. L. (2000). Self-determination theory and the facilitation of intrinsic motivation, social development, and well-being. *American Psychologist, 55*(1), 68–78. doi:10.1037/0003-066X.55.1.68

Sabogal, F., Marin, G., Otero-Sabogal, R., Marin, B. V., & Perez-Stable, E. J. (1987). Hispanic familism and acculturation: What changes and what doesn't? *Hispanic Journal of Behavioural Sciences, 9*(4), 397–412. doi:10.1177/07399863870094003

Salter, K., Zettler, L., Foley, N., & Teasell, R. (2010). Impact of caring for individuals with stroke on perceived physical health of informal caregivers. *Disability Rehabilitation, 32*(4), 273–281. doi:10.3109/09638280903114394

Sands, L. P., Ferreira, P., Stewart, A. L., Brod, M., & Yaffe, K. (2004). What explains differences between dementia patients' and their caregivers' ratings of patients' quality of life? *American Journal of Geriatric Psychiatry, 12*(3), 272–280. doi:10.1097/00019442-200405000-00006

Savundranayagam, M. Y., & Montgomery, R. J. (2013). Profile of the caregiving career: Do experiences of burden and depression differ among spouses and adult-children? *Psychology & Health, 28*, 53 (Abstract).

Savundranayagam, M. Y., Montgomery, R. J., & Kosloski, K. (2011). A dimensional analysis of caregiver burden among spouses and adult children. *The Gerontologist, 51*(3), 321–331. doi:10.1093/geront/gnq102

Schmall, V. L. (1995). Family caregiver education and training: Enhancing self-efficacy. *Journal of Case Management, 4*, 156–162.

Schulz, R., & Beach, S. (1999). Caregiving as a risk factor for mortality. *Journal of the American Medical Association, 282*(23), 2215–2219. doi:10.1001/jama.282.23.2215

Schulz, R., Belle, S. H., Czaja, S. J., McGinnis, K. A., Stevens, A., & Zhang, S. (2004). Long-term care placement of dementia patients and caregiver health and well-being. *Journal of the American Medical Association, 292*(8), 961–967. doi:10.1001/jama.292.8.961

Schulz, R., Boerner, K., Shear, K., Zhang, S., & Gitlin, L. N. (2006). Predictors of complicated grief among dementia caregivers: A prospective study of bereavement. *American Journal of Geriatric Psychiatry, 14*(8), 650–658. doi:10.1097/01.JGP.0000203178.44894.db

Schulz, R., & Martire, L. M. (2004). Family caregiving of persons with dementia: Prevalence, health effects and support strategies. *American Journal of Geriatric Psychiatry, 12*, 240–249. doi:10.1097/00019442-200405000-00002

Schulz, R. & Patterson, T. L. (2004). Caregiving in geriatric psychiatry (Editorial). *American Journal of Geriatric Psychiatry, 12*, 234–37. doi.org/10.1176/appi.ajgp.12.3.234

Schulz, R., Rosen, J., Klinger, J., Musa, D., Castle, N. G., Kane, A. L., & Lustig, A. (2014). Effects of a psychosocial intervention on caregivers of recently placed nursing home residents: A randomized controlled trial. *Clinical Gerontologist, 37*, 347–367. doi:10.1080/07317115.2014.907594

Shaver, P. R., & Mikulincer, M. (Eds.). (2008). *A behavioral systems perspective on prosocial behavior: Prosocial motives, emotions, and behavior*. Washington, DC: APA. doi:10.1037/12061-000

Shaw, W. S., Patterson, T. L., Semple, S. J., Dimsdale, J. E., Ziegler, M. G., & Grant, I. (2003). Emotional expressiveness, hostility and blood pressure in a longitudinal cohort of Alzheimer caregivers. *Journal of Psychosomatic Research, 54*(4), 293–302. doi:10.1016/S0022-3999(02)00412-9

Sherman, D. W., McGuire, D. B., Free, D., &, Cheon, J. Y. (2014). A pilot study of the experience of family caregivers of patients with advanced pancreatic cancer using a mixed methods approach. *Journal of Pain and Symptom Management, 48*(3), 385–399. doi:10.1016/j.jpainsymman.2013.09.006

Shields, A., Park, M., Ward, S. E., & Song, M. (2010). Subject recruitment and retention against quadruple challenges in an intervention trial of end-of-life communication. *Journal of Hospice & Palliative Nursing, 12*(5), 312–318. doi:10.1097/NJH.0b013e3181ec9dd1

Shumaker, S. A., & Hill, D. R. (1991). Gender differences in social support and physical health. *Health Psychology, 10*(2), 102–111. doi:10.1037/0278-6133.10.2.102

Shurgot, G. R., & Knight, B. G. (2005). Influence of neuroticism, ethnicity, familism, and social support on perceived burden in dementia caregivers: Pilot test of the transactional stress and social support model. *The Journals of Gerontology Series B: Psychological Sciences and Social Sciences of Gerontology, 60,* 331–334. doi:10.1093/geronb/60.6.P331

Silverman, M. (2013). Sighs, smiles, and worried glances: How the body reveals women caregivers' lived experiences of care to older adults. *Journal of Aging Studies, 27*(3), 288–297. doi:10.1016/j.jaging.2013.06.001

Silverman, M. (2015). Observing women caregivers' everyday experiences: New ways of understanding and intervening. *Journal of Gerontological Social Work, 58*(2), 206–222. doi:10.1080/01634372.2014.939384

Simon, C., Kumar, S., Kendrick, T. (2008). Formal support of stroke survivors and their informal carers in the community: A cohort study. *Health Social Care Community, 16*(6), 582–92. doi:10.1111/j.1365-2524.2008.00782

Skaff, M. M., Pearlin, L. I., & Mullan, J. T. (1996). Transitions in the caregiving career: Effects on sense of mastery. *Psychology & Aging, 11,* 247–257. doi:10.1037/0882-7974.11.2.247

Smith, T. W., Gallo, L. C., Shivpuri, S., & Brewer, A. L. (2012). Personality and health: Current issues and emerging perspectives. In A. Baum, T. A. Revenson, & J. Singer (Eds.), *Handbook of health psychology*, 2nd edition (pp. 374–404). New York: Taylor & Francis.

Smith, T. W., Williams, P. G., & Segerstrom, S. C. (2015). Personality and physical health. In M. Mikulincer & P. R. Shaver (Eds.), *Handbook of personality and social psychology: Vol. 4, Personality processes and individual differences* (pp. 639–661). Washington, DC: American Psychological Association.

Sneeuw, K., Aaronson, N., Sprangers, M., Detmar, S., Wever, L., & Schornagel, J. (1998). Comparison of patient and proxy EORTC QLQ-C30 ratings in assessing the quality of life of cancer patients. *Journal of Clinical Epidemiology, 51*(7), 617–631. doi:10.1016/S0895-4356(98)00040-7

Sneeuw, K., Sprangers, M., & Aaronson, N. (2002). The role of health care providers and significant others in evaluating the quality of life of patients with chronic disease. *Journal of Clinical Epidemiology, 55*(11), 1130–1143. doi:10.1016/S0895-4356(02)00479-1

Sörensen, S., Pinquart, M., & Duberstein, P. (2002). How effective are interventions with caregivers? An updated meta-analysis. *The Gerontologist, 42,* 356–372. doi:10.1093/geront/42.3.356

Soskolne, V., Halevy-Levin, S., Cohen, A., & Friedman, G. (2006). Caregiving stressors and psychological distress among veteran resident and immigrant family caregivers in Israel. *Social Work in Health Care, 43*(2–3), 73–93. doi:10.1300/J010v43n02_06

Spencer-Rodgers, J., Williams, M. J., & Peng, K. (2010). Cultural differences in expectations of change and tolerance for contradiction: A decade of empirical research. *Personality & Social Psychology Review, 14*(3), 296–312. doi:10.1177/1088868310362982

Spillers, R. L., Wellisch, D. K., Kim, Y., Matthews, A., & Baker, F. (2008). Family caregivers and guilt in the context of cancer care. *Psychosomatics, 49*(6), 511–519. doi:10.1176/appi.psy.49.6.511

Stajduhar, K. I., Funk, L., Toye, C., Grande, G. E., Aoun, S., & Todd, C. J. (2010). Part 1: Home-based family caregiving at the end of life: A comprehensive review of published quantitative research (1998–2008). *Palliative Medicine, 24*(6), 573–593. doi:10.1177/0269216310371412

Stanton, A., Revenson, T. A., & Tennen, H. (2007). Health psychology: Psychological adjustment to chronic disease. *Annual Review of Psychology, 58,* 13.1–13.28. doi: 10.1146/annurev.psych.58.110405.085615

Stanton, A. L., Danoff-Burg, S., Cameron, C. L., & Ellis, A. P. (1994). Coping through emotional approach: Problems of conceptualizaton and confounding. *Journal of Personality and Social Psychology, 66*(2), 350–362. doi:10.1037/0022-3514.66.2.350.

Steel, P., Schmidt, J., & Shultz, J. (2008). Refining the relationship between personality and subjective well-being. *Psychological Bulletin, 134,* 138–161. doi.org/10.1037/0033-2909.134.1.138

Stromberg, A., & Luttik, M. L. (2015). Burden of caring: Risks and consequences imposed on caregivers of those living and dying with advanced heart failure. *Current Opinion on Support and Palliative Care, 9*(1), 26–30. doi:10.1097/SPC.0000000000000111

Suls, J., Green, P., Rose, G., Lounsbury, P., & Gordon, E. (1997). Hiding worries from one's spouse: Associations between coping via protective buffering and distress in male post-myocardial infarction patients and their wives. *Journal of Behavioral Medicine, 20*(4), 333–349. doi:10.1023/A:1025513029605

Tang, Y. (2006). Obligation of filial piety, adult child caregiver burden, *received social support and psychological wellbeing of adult child caregivers for frail elderly in Guangzhou, China* (Unpublished doctoral dissertation). The University of Hong Kong, Hong Kong.

Tang, S., Liu, T., Lai, M., Liu, L., & Chen, C. (2005). Concordance of preferences for end-of-life care between terminally ill cancer patients and their family caregivers in Taiwan. *Journal of Pain and Symptom Management, 30*(6), 510–518. doi:10.1016/j.jpainsymman.2005.05.019

Taylor, S. E., Klein, L. C., Lewis, B. P., Gruenewald, T. L., Gurung, R. A., & Updegraff, J. A. (2000). Biobehavioral responses to stress in females: Tend-and-befriend, not fight-or-flight. *Psychological Review, 107*(3), 411. doi:10.1037/0033-295X.107.3.411

The Economist Intelligence Unit Limited (2011). Future of Healthcare in Europe. http://www.janssen-emea.com/sites/default/files/The-Future-Of-Healthcare-In-Europe.pdf. Retrieved July 13, 2105.

Thomsen, D. K., Jørgensen, M. M., Mehlsen, M. Y., & Zachariae, R. (2004). The influence of rumination and defensiveness on negative affect in response to experimental stress. *Scandinavian Journal of Psychology, 45*(3), 253–258. doi:10.1111/j.1467-9450.2004.00402.x

Tiedens, L. Z., & Leach, C. W. (2004). *The social life of emotions.* New York: Cambridge University Press.

Tokem, Y., Ozcelik, H., & Cicik, A. (2015). Examination of the relationship between hopelessness levels and coping strategies among the family caregivers of patients with cancer. *Cancer Nursing, 38*(4), 28–34. doi:10.1097/NCC.0000000000000189

Tong, A., Sainsbury, P., & Craig, J. C. (2008). Support interventions for caregivers of people with chronic kidney disease: A systematic review. *Nephrology, Dialysis, & Transplantation, 23*, 3960–3965. doi:10.1093/ndt/gfn415

Traa, M. J., De Vries, J., Bodenmann, G., & Den Oudsten, B. L. (2015). Dyadic coping and relationship functioning in couples coping with cancer: A systematic review. *British Journal of Health Psychology, 20*(1), 85–114. doi:10.1111/bjhp.12094

Trail, M., Nelson, N., Van, J. N., Appel, S. H., & Lai, E. C. (2004). Major stressors facing patients with amyotrophic lateral sclerosis (ALS): A survey to identify their concerns and to compare with those of their caregivers. *Amyotrophic Lateral Sclerosis and Other Motor Neuron Disorders, 5*(1), 40–45. doi:10.1080/14660820310016075

Travis, S. S., Bernard, M. A., McAuley, W. J., Thornton, M., & Kole, T. (2003). Development of the family caregiver medication administration hassles scale. *The Gerontologist, 43*(3), 360–368. doi:10.1093/geront/43.3.360

Triantafillou, J., Naiditch, M., Repkova, K., Stiehr, K., Carretero, S., Emilsson, T., DiSanto, P., Bednarik, R., Brichtova, L., Ceruzzi, F., Cordero, L., Mastroyiannakis, T., Ferrando, M., Mingot, M., Ritter, J., & Vlantoni, D. (2010). Informal care in the long-term system. European Overview Paper. Interlinks: Athens/Vienna. http://www.euro.centre.org/data/1278594816_84909.pdf. Retrieved January 12, 2015.

Trotter, R. T. (2001). Curanderismo: A picture of Mexican-American folk healing. *Journal of Alternative and Complementary Medicine, 7*(2), 129–131. doi:10.1089/107555301750164163

Trudeau, K. J., Danoff-Burg, S., Revenson, T. A., & Paget, S. A. (2003). Agency and communion in people with rheumatoid arthritis. *Sex Roles, 49*(7–8), 303–311. doi:10.1023/A:1025192818638

Tsai, P. C., Yip, P. K., Tai, J. J., & Lou, M. F. (2015). Needs of family caregivers of stroke patients: A longitudinal study of caregivers' perspectives. *Patient Preference and Adherence, 9*, 449–457. doi:10.2147/PPA.S77713

Tsilika, E., Parpa, E., Zygogianni, A., Kouloulias, V., & Mystakidou, K. (2014). Caregivers' attachment patterns and their interactions with cancer patients' patterns. *Supportive Care in Cancer, 23*, 87–94. doi:10.1007/s00520-014-2329-6

Ugur, O., & Fadiloglu, C. (2010). Caregiver Strain Index: Validity and reliability in Turkish society. *Asian Pacific Journal of Cancer Prevention, 11*, 1669–1675.

United Nations (2003). Convention on the elimination of all forms of discrimination against women [online]. http://www.un.org/womenwatch/daw/cedaw/text/econvention.htm. Retrieved March 15, 2012.

Ussher, J. M., & Perz, J. (2010). Gender differences in self-silencing and psychological distress in informal cancer carers. *Psychology of Women Quarterly, 34*(2), 228–242. doi: 10.1111/j.1471-6402.2010.01564.x

Välimäki, T., Martikainen, J., Hongisto, K., Fraunberg, M., Hallikainen, I., Sivenius, J., Vehvilainen-Julkunen, K., Pietila, A. M., Koivisto, A. M., & ALSOVA Study Group (2014). Decreasing sense of coherence and its determinants in spousal caregivers of persons with mild Alzheimer's disease in three year follow-up: ALSOVA study. *International Psychogeriatrics, 26*, 1211–1220. doi:/10.1017/S1041610214000428

Van Assche, L., Luyten, P., Bruffaerts, R., Persoons, P., van de Ven, L., & Vandenbulcke, M. (2013). Attachment in old age: Theoretical assumptions, empirical findings and implications for clinical practice. *Clinical Psychology Review, 33*, 67–81. doi:10.1016/j.cpr.2012.10.003

van den Heuvel, E. T., de Witte, L. P., Schure, L. M., Sanderman, R., & Meyboom-de Jong, B. (2001). Risk factors for burn-out in caregivers of stroke patients, and possibilities for intervention. *Clinical Rehabilitation, 15*(6), 669–677. doi:10.1191/0269215501cr446oa

Van Exel, N. J., Brouwer, W. B., Van den Berg, B., Koopmanschap, M. A., & Van den Bos, G. A. (2004). What really matters: An inquiry into the relative importance of dimensions of informal caregiver burden. *Clinical Rehabilitation, 18*(6), 683–693. doi:10.1191/0269215504cr7430a

van Ryn, M., Sanders, S., Kahn, K., van Houtven, C., Griffin, J. M., Martin, M., Atienza, A. A., Phelan, S., Finstad, D., & Rowland, J. (2011). Objective burden, resources, and other stressors among informal cancer caregivers: A hidden quality issue? *Psycho-Oncology, 20*(1), 44–52. doi:10.1002/pon.1703

VanYperen, N., & Buunk, B. (1990). A longitudinal-study of equity and satisfaction in intimate-relationships. *European Journal of Social Psychology, 20*(4), 287–309. doi:10.1002/ejsp.2420200403

Vaughn, L. M., Jacquez, F., & Baker, R. C. (2009). Cultural health attributions, beliefs, and practices: Effects on healthcare and medical education. *The Open Medical Education Journal, 2*, 64–74. http://benthamopen.com/ABSTRACT/TOMEDEDUJ-2-16

Vedhara, K., Shanks, N., Wilcock, G., & Lightman, S. L. (2001). Correlates and predictors of self-reported psychological and physical morbidity in chronic caregiver stress. *Journal of Health Psychology, 6*, 101–119. doi:10.1177/135910530100600108

Vilchinsky, N., Dekel, R., Leibowitz, M., Reges, O., Khaskia, A., & Mosseri, M. (2011). Dynamics of support perceptions among couples coping with cardiac illness: The effect on recovery outcomes. *Health Psychology, 30*(4), 411–419. doi:10.1037/a0023453

Vilchinsky, N., Dekel, R., Revenson, T. A., Liberman, G., & Mosseri, M. (2015(. Caregiver burden and depressive symptoms: The moderational role of attachment orientations. *Health Psychology, 34*, 262–269. doi:10.1037/hea0000121

Vilchinsky, N., Haze-Filderman, L., Leibowitz, M., Reges, O., Khaskia, A., & Mosseri, M. (2010). Spousal support and cardiac patients' distress: The moderating role of attachment orientation. *Journal of Family Psychology, 24*, 508–512. doi:10.1037/a0020009

Vitaliano, P. P., Young, H. M., & Zhang, J. (2004). Is caregiving a risk factor for illness? *Current Directions in Psychological Science, 13*(1), 13–16. doi:10.1111/j.0963-7214.2004.01301004.x

Vitaliano, P. P., Zhang, J., & Scanlan, J. M. (2003). Is caregiving hazardous to one's physical health? A meta-analysis. *Psychological Bulletin, 129*(6), 946–972. doi:10.1037/0033-2909.129.6.946

Waldron, E. A., Janke, E. A., Bechtel, C. F., Ramirez, M., & Cohen, A. (2013). A systematic review of psychosocial interventions to improve cancer caregiver quality of life. *Psycho-Oncology, 22*, 1200–1207. doi:10.1002/pon.3118

Walker, A. J., Pratt, C. C., Shin, H. Y., & Jones, L. L. (1990). Motives for parental caregiving and relationship quality. *Family Relations, 39*(1), 51–56. doi:10.2307/584948

Walker, R. C., Hanson, C. S., Palmer, S. C., Howard, K., Morton, R. L., Marshall, M. R., & Tong, A. (2015). Patient and caregiver perspectives on home hemodialysis: A systematic review. *American Journal of Kidney Diseases, 65*(3), 451–463. doi:10.1053/j.ajkd.2014.10.020

Walster, E., & Berscheid, E. (1973). New directions in equity research. *Journal of Personality and Social Psychology, 25*(2), 151–176. doi:10.1037/h0033967

Weitzner, M. A., Jacobsen, P. B., Wagner H., Friedland, J., & Cox, C. (1999). The Caregiver Quality of Life Index–Cancer (CQOLC) scale: Development and validation of an instrument to measure quality of life of the family caregiver of patients with cancer. *Quality of Life Research, 8* (1–2), 55–63. doi:10.1023/A:1026407010614

Whitlatch, C., Feinberg, L., & Tucke, S. (2005). Measuring the values and preferences for everyday care of persons with cognitive impairment and their family caregivers. *The Gerontologist, 45*(3), 370–380. doi:10.1093/geront/45.3.370

Whittingham, K., Barnes, S., & Gardiner, C. (2013). Tools to measure quality of life and carer burden in informal carers of heart failure patients: A narrative review. *Palliative Medicine, 27*(7), 596–607. doi:10.1177/0269216313477179

Williams, A. L., Tisch, A. J. H., Dixon, J., & McCorkle, R. (2013). Factors associated with depressive symptoms in cancer family caregivers of patients receiving chemotherapy. *Supportive Care in Cancer, 21*(9), 2387–2394. doi:10.1007/s00520-013-1802-y

Williams, K. L., Morrison, V., & Robinson, C. A. (2014). Exploring caregiving experiences: Caregiver coping and making sense of illness. *Aging & Mental Health, 18*(5), 600–609. doi:10.1080/13607863.2013.860425

Williams, V. P., Bishop-Fitzpatrick, L., Lane, J. D., Gwyther, L. P., Ballard, E. L., Vendittelli, A. P., Hutchins, T. S., & Williams, R. B. (2010). Video-based coping skills to reduce health risk and improve psychological and physical well-being in Alzheimer's disease family caregivers. *Psychosomatic Medicine, 72*(9), 897–904. doi:10.1097/PSY.0b013e3181fc2d09

Wolff J. L., & Kasper J. D. (2006). Caregivers of frail elders: Updating a national profile. *The Gerontologist, 46*, 344–356. doi:10.1093/geront/46.3.344

Wolff, J. L., & Roter, D. L. (2011). Family presence in routine medical visits: A meta-analytical review. *Social Science & Medicine, 72*, 823–831. doi:10.1001/jama.2012.13366

Yaffe, K., Fox, P., Newcomer, R., Sands, L., Lindquist, K., Dane, K., & Covinsky, K. E. (2002). Patient and caregiver characteristics and nursing home placement in patients with dementia. *Journal of the American Medical Association, 287*(16), 2090–2097. doi:10.1001/jama.287.16.2090

Yates, M. E., Tennstedt, S., & Chang, B. H. (1999). Contributors to and mediators of psychological well-being for informal caregivers. *The Journals of Gerontology Series B: Psychological Sciences and Social Sciences, 54*(1), 12–22. doi:10.1093/geronb/54B.1.P12

Yee, J. L., & Schulz, R. (2000). Gender differences in psychiatric morbidity among family caregivers a review and analysis. *The Gerontologist, 40*(2), 147–164. doi:10.1093/geront/40.2.147

Ybema, J., Kuijer, R., Buunk, B., DeJong, G., & Sanderman, R. (2001). Depression and perceptions of inequity among couples facing cancer. *Personality and Social Psychology Bulletin, 27*(1), 3–13. doi:10.1177/0146167201271001

Youn, G., Knight, B. G., Jeong, H. S., & Benton, D. (1999). Differences in familism values and caregiving outcomes among Korean, Korean-American, and White-American dementia caregivers. *Psychology & Aging, 14*(3), 355–364. doi:10.1037/0882-7974.14.3.355

Zarit, S. H., & Reamy, A. M. (2013). Future directions in family and professional caregiving for the elderly. *Gerontology, 59*(2), 152–158. doi:10.1159/000342242

Zarit, S. H., Reever, K. E., & Bach-Peterson, J. (1980). Relatives of the impaired elderly: Correlates of feelings of burden. *The Gerontologist, 20*(6), 649–655. doi:10.1093/geront/20.6.649

Zarit, S. H., Todd, P. A., & Zarit, J. M. (1986). Subjective burden of husbands and wives as caregivers: A longitudinal study. *The Gerontologist, 26*, 260–266. doi:10.1093/geront/26.3.260

Zhang, A., & Siminoff, L. (2003). Silence and cancer: Why do families and patients fail to communicate? *Health Communication, 15*(4), 415–429. doi:10.1207/S15327027HC1504_03

Zunkel, G. (2003). Relational coping processes: Couples' response to a diagnosis of early stage breast cancer. *Journal of Psychosocial Oncology, 20*(4), 39–55. doi:10.1300/J077v20n04_03

Index

Note: 'f' indicates figure, 't' indicates table

adaptation hypothesis, 21
adult children, 27, 34, 55, 59, 60, 61, 68–69, 71, 76
   daughters, 50, 60–62, 68, 70, 75
   sons, 60–62, 68
agency, 56
   see also unmitigated agency
agreeableness, 81, 84, 86, 87, 88
Alzheimer's disease, 43, 44, 85, 87
anger, 39, 43, 44, 76, 84
Antonovsky, A., 83, 106
anxiety, 18, 40, 43, 47, 74–75, 76, 82, 84–85, 86, 88, 89, 92, 94, 96, 97–98, 104
appraisal
   of caregiving, 11, 12, 13, 23
   of illness, 27, 84
   of stress, cognitive, 8–10, 52, 56, 83
attachment anxiety, 82, 84–85, 86
attachment avoidance, 82, 84–85, 87, 89
attachment orientations, 11, 80, 82–83, 88
attachment security, 82, 84, 86–87
attachment theory, 82

Badr, H., 18, 29, 30, 95

Bakas Caregiving Outcomes Scale (BCOS), 23–24
Berg, C. A., 9, 27, 29
Bookwala, J., 81, 83, 84, 85, 86
Bowlby, J., 82
Buckwalter, K. C., 51, 54, 55, 56, 58, 60, 62
burden, 7, 13, 26, 41, 43, 47, 49, 54–57, 59–61, 63, 65, 68, 76, 77, 83, 86, 88, 91–94, 97–98, 100, 102
   and activity restriction, 17–18
   and familism, 71
   and gender differences, 50–54
   and hiding one's feelings, 30, 31, 33
   and illness trajectory, 4, 12, 17–19, 44
   measures of, 22–24, 23t
   objective, 3, 9, 16–17, 21, 35, 52–53
   subjective, 9, 17, 22, 23, 52–53

cancer
   brain, 98
   breast, 29, 30, 31, 55, 57
   colorectal, 28, 51
   lung, 30, 31
   pancreatic, 5
   prostate, 29, 30, 93
   terminal, 34–35

Index

cancer caregivers, 3, 4–5, 7, 17, 21–22, 23, 28, 42–44, 51, 55, 60, 86, 104
care recipient(s), 2, 14, 39, 53, 55, 70, 71, 74, 75, 78, 91, 93
   and caregiver support, 6, 21, 27–29
   and emotions, 43–47
   life ratings of, 33–34
   and personality, 80, 85, 87–89
   relationship between caregiver and, 9–12, 18–20, 22, 28–29, 32, 34, 41, 46, 50, 59–62
caregiver dyads, 12, 26, 27–37, *see also* dyadic coping
Caregiver Reaction Assessment (CRA), 23
caregiver(s)
   adjustment to the role, 85–87
   adult children as, 27, 34, 55, 59, 60, 61, 68–69, 71, 76
   of Alzheimer's disease, 43, 44, 85, 87
   Asian Indian, 70–71
   British South Asian (BSA), 70, 74–75, 77
   burden, *see* burden
   Canadian, 54, 71
   cancer, *see* cancer caregivers
   and care recipient, *see* care recipient(s)
   Caribbean, 55–56
   Chinese, 77
   core individual values and responses of, 70–71
   daughters as, 50, 60–62, 68, 70, 75
   daughters-in-law as, 50, 68, 72, 75
   dementia, *see* dementia caregivers
   East Asian, 72–73
   emotions of, *see* emotions
   ethnic minority, 65, 69, 71–72, 76, 77
   family, *see* family caregivers
   female, 3, 18, 42, 44, 49, 50, 53, 56, 57, 58–59, 61, 75, 86, *see also* women caregivers
   health of, 2, 3, 4–5, 18–20, 42, 45–46, 57, 85–87, *see also* well-being of caregivers
   Hispanic, 67, 71, 74
   informal, *see* family caregivers
   interventions for, *see* interventions
   Korean, 74, 76
   Latino, 55–56, 62, 71, 76
   male, 42, 49, 50, 53, 55, 59, 62, 87
   non-Hispanic White, 65, 71, 76
   non-primary, 3
   North American Indian, 73
   older/elderly, 20, 77
   primary, 3, 60, 104
   sibling, 7, 50, 60, 72
   spouses as, *see* spousal caregiving
   stress, *see* stress
   of stroke patients, 92, 93, 97–99, 101
   tasks of, 5–6
   Thai, 76, 102
   unpaid, 3, 5, 14, 53, 59
   well-being, *see* well-being of caregivers
   White, 55, 65, 71, 76
   White-British (WB), 70, 71, 74–75, 77
   see also caregiving
Caregiver Strain Index (CSI), 23
caregiver stress and appraisal model, 9
caregiver stress process model, 9
caregiving
   and cultural influence, 10, 12, 19, 27, 51, 61, *see also* culture and caregiving
   definition of, 5
   as a dyadic process, *see* dyadic coping
   economic value of, 14
   employment patterns and, 54
   in the end-of-life phase, 31, 34–37, 94–97, 102
   family, *see* family caregivers
   framework for study of, 10–13, 10f
   gender and, *see* gender and caregiving
   impact on caregiver's health, 2, 3, 4–5, 18–20, 42, 45–46, 57, 85–87, *see also* well-being of caregivers
   informal, 2–7, 21, 24, 65, 67, 69, 78
   issues at a dyadic level, 33–35

caregiving – *Continued*
  measurement of, 7–8
  models of, 8–10
  motivations for, *see* motivations/
    motives
  negative aspects of, 70, 76–77
  outcomes, *see* outcomes of
    caregiving
  personality and, *see* personality and
    caregiving
  positive aspects of, 77
  statistics, 2–5, 69
  stress, 13, 16, 17, 18, 19, 21–24, 46, 49,
    74, 75, 76
  time spent on, 3–5
  transformative, 21
  versus social support, 6–7
  see also caregiver(s)
Carmack, C. L., 18, 29, 95
Carver, C. S., 5, 22, 40, 51, 83, 84
change principle, 72
Chi, N-C., 94, 97–103
China, 65, 68, 71
chronic illness, 2, 4, 10, 11, 12, 26, 27, 37,
  49, 50, 68, 80, 91, 93, 95, 97–100
collectivism, 67, 76
communication, 27, 29–33, 37, 88,
  93–95, 103, 104
communion, 56
  see also unmitigated communion
conscientiousness, 81, 84, 86, 87
contradiction principle, 72
COPE framework, 94
coping, 56–59, 65, 76, 80, 85, 86, 94–95,
  100, 103, 104
  behavior, 10, 12, 27, 73
  collaborative, 27, 29, 37
  as a couple, 26–30, 53, 55, 56, 62, 86,
    97, 98
  emotional labor, 44
  emotion-focused, 42, 43
  emotions as strategy for, 42–45, 47, 51
  with hope, 44–45
  models, 8–10
  problem-focused, 42–43
  process, 27, 44, 58

religious, 70, 77
resources, 9, 11
strategies, 39, 41, 42–45, 47, 51, 58,
  70, 88, 94
stress and, 8–9, 42–44, 63, 65, 67,
  73, 83
see also dyadic coping
couples, 10, 26–32, 36–37, 42, 49, 53, 55,
  56, 59, 62, 86, 93, 97, 98
see also dyad; dyadic coping
culture, 10, 12, 19, 27, 51, 61, 65–66
culture and caregiving
  age of caregivers, 71–72
  caregivers' experience, 75–76
  collectivism and individualism, 67
  core individual values and caregiver
    responses, 70–71
  future research, 78
  gender roles, 72
  governmental policies, 67–68
  negative aspects of caregiving, 70,
    76–77
  perceptions of illness, 72–74
  positive aspects of caregiving, 77
  social expectancies of care, 68–69

death, 4, 18, 31, 32, 34, 46, 47, 93
dementia caregivers, 4, 12, 17, 19, 22, 23,
  32, 34, 35, 37, 42, 46, 50, 61, 78, 84,
  85, 87
depression, 4–5, 7, 9, 11, 18, 19, 26, 28,
  32, 43, 45, 47, 51, 57, 58, 60, 75, 76,
  85, 87, 92, 94, 96, 97–98, 100, 104
developmental–contextual model of
  dyadic coping, 9–10, 27
dispositional optimism, 83
distress, 3, 16, 27, 29, 30–33, 36, 40–43,
  55, 57–59, 63, 76, 88, 89, 97, 100
  emotional, 18–19, 41, 45–46, 50, 52,
    58
  psychological, 2, 4, 9, 18, 20, 22, 42,
    86
dyad, 9–10, 11, 12, 13, 14, 26–27, 29,
  31, 32, 33, 35–37, 50, 55, 87, 95, 96,
  97–102
see also dyadic coping

dyadic coping, 9–10, 26–27, 55, 95
  collaborative coping, 27, 29, 37
  communication and intimacy processes, 29–33
  exchange of support, 27–29
  limitations and future research, 35–37
  perspectives on formal care, 34–35
  ratings on patients' quality of life, 33–34
  recruitment of dyads, 36–37
  research, 27, 35–37

elderly, caregiving for, 2–4, 11–12, 22, 23, 27, 34, 37, 44, 50, 59, 60, 62, 65, 68, 74, 77, 92
emotional disclosure, 29–32, 57–58
emotional distress, *see* distress, emotional
emotional labor, 44
emotional preparedness, 47, 92–93, 96
emotional recovery, 46–47
emotional support, 6, 7, 26, 28–29, 33, 58, 59
emotions, 10, 13, 30, 31, 32, 51, 56, 58, 62, 81, 85
  as coping strategies, 42–45
  as motivations, 39–42, *see also* motivations/motives
  as outcomes, 45–47
  see also anger; anxiety; frustration; guilt; shame
empathic concern, 40
empathic distress, 40
empathy-altruism hypothesis, 40
ethnicity, 66, 78
EUROFAMCARE study, 68, 77, 78
exhaustion, 20, 44, 57, 59
extraversion, 81, 84, 86

familism, 19, 70–71, 76–77
family caregivers, 2–5, 7, 14, 20, 22, 34, 41, 43, 44, 45, 52, 54, 59–62, 84, 99, 102

female caregivers, 3, 13, 18, 20, 32, 42, 44, 46, 49–50, 61, 75, 86
Feinberg, L., 14, 35, 49
filial obligation, 68, 70, 71
filial piety, 70, 71, 77
filial responsibility, *see* filial piety
five-factor model of personality, 80, 81, 85
Folkman, S., 8, 9, 42, 43, 83
Friedemann, M. L., 50, 54, 55, 56, 58, 60, 62
frustration, 39, 44, 77

gender and caregiving
  amount of care, 52–54
  employment patterns, 54
  future directions, 62
  gender roles, 52, 72
  motivations for caregiving, 54–56
  relationship of caregiver to patient, 59–62
  statistics, 49–50, 59–60
  stress and burden, 50–54
  women and interpersonal relationships, 56–59
guilt, 19, 39, 40, 41, 45, 46, 60, 74, 84

Hagedoorn, M., 8, 12, 27, 30, 36, 37, 49, 50, 52, 57, 58, 61, 88
hardiness, 83
holism, 72–73
hospice care, 33, 35, 44, 96, 102, 103
  see also institutionalization

illness trajectory, 4, 12, 17, 18, 43, 51, 60, 96, 104
individualism, 67
informal caregiving, 2–7, 21, 24, 65, 67, 69, 78
informal caregivers, *see* family caregivers
institutionalization, 16, 19, 41, 46, 91
  see also hospice care
instrumental support, 6, 28, 29, 59, 76
interpersonal process model, 30

interventions, 13, 14, 24, 26, 30, 36, 43–44, 47, 78, 88
  and caregiver burden, 97–98
  competence and mastery of caregivers, 98–99
  cultural issues in, 102–103
  delivery of, 100–101
  effectiveness of, 96–98
  feasibility and reach with, 101–102
  future research directions, 103–104
  information and educational, 92–93, 98
  limitations of research, 99–100
  physical health of caregivers, 99
  practical support, respite services, 91–92
  psychosocial support, 93–95
  quality of life (QOL) of caregivers, 97
  self-care, 95–96
  social and family functioning of caregivers, 98
intimacy, 6, 1, 27, 28, 29–33, 37, 45, 52, 61, 74

Lazarus, R. S., 8, 9, 42, 43, 83
Leventhal, H., 12, 73, 93

male caregivers, 42, 49, 63, 87
  employment patterns, 54
  motivations for caregiving, 54–56
  relationship of caregiver to patient, 59–62
  stress and burden, 50–54
  unmitigated agency, 57
mastery, 83, 86, 87, 88, 92, 98–99, 104
Morrison, V., 21, 68, 70, 71, 77
Motivations in Elder Caregiving Scale, 74
motivations/motives, 13, 31, 57, 62
  for caregiving, 54–56, 74–75
  dimensions of, 41
  emotions as, 39–42, 47
  external, 40
  extrinsic, 41, 74, 75
  frameworks for caregiver, 40–41
  integrated, 40, 41
  intrinsic, 41, 74, 75
  introjected, 40–41, 84
  measures for, 74–75
  obligation-based, 41, 55
  personal, 41
  personality and, 84–85
  relation to caregiver outcomes, 41–42

neuroticism, 81, 84, 85, 86, 87, 88

objective burden, 3, 9, 16–17, 35, 52–53
openness, 81, 84, 87
outcomes of caregiving, 7, 8–11, 13
  emotions and, 45–47
  measures of, 22–24, 23t
  mental health, 18–19, 85–86
  negative, 9, 11, 18–19, 43, 45, 47, 81, 87
  over time, 21–22
  personality and, see personality and caregiving
  physical health, 20, 87
  positive, 11, 20–21, 23, 41, 45, 86–87
  relation of motivations to, 41–42

palliative care, see hospice care
Parkinson's disease, 12, 17, 85
Parveen, S., 21, 68, 70, 71, 74–77
patient(s), see care recipient(s)
Pearlin, L. I., 5, 6, 9, 22, 39, 83
personality and caregiving, 8, 11, 13, 46, 56, 59, 80–81
  adjustment to the caregiver role, 85–87
  attachment orientations, 80, 82–83, 88
  five-factor model of personality, 81
  motivation and ability, 84–85
  social support and care acceptance, 87–88
  stress-resistance resources, 83
Pinquart, M., 11, 16, 21, 49, 50, 51, 52, 60, 63, 65, 67, 68, 71, 76, 100

protective buffering, 31, 58
psychological distress, *see* distress, psychological

quality of life (QOL), 33–34, 40, 44, 77, 92, 94, 96, 97, 100, 104

randomized controlled trials (RCTs), 91–92, 96, 97, 98, 100
respite care, 19, 54, 91–92, 96, 104
Revenson, T. A., 8, 12, 18, 19, 21, 29, 50, 52, 53, 57, 58, 59, 63, 80, 87, 95
rheumatoid arthritis, 17, 49, 53, 57, 59
role overload, 9, 60

salutogenic effects of caregiving, 83
Schulz, R., 81, 83, 84, 85, 86
self-determination theory, 40–41
self-esteem, 28, 29, 52, 55, 61, 63, 86
self-regulation theory, 83, 94
sense of coherence (SOC), 83, 86
shame, 39, 41, 46, 84
Shaver, P. R., 80, 82, 83, 84, 88
social support, 6–7, 27, 34, 45, 56, 57–58, 76, 81, 87–88, 94, 98, 104
Sörensen, S., 11, 16, 21, 49, 50, 51, 52, 60, 63, 65, 67, 68, 71, 76, 100
spousal caregiving, 3, 7, 19, 26, 28, 29–30, 31, 34, 37, 42, 46, 49, 53, 55, 58–61, 68–69, 71–72, 76
stress, 2, 4–6, 88
  caregiving, 13, 16, 17, 18, 19, 21–24, 46, 49, 74, 75, 76
  coping and, 8–9, 42–44, 63, 65, 67, 73, 83
  -diathesis model, 81
  and gender differences, 50–55, 56, 58, 59, 61
  interventions for reduction of, 92, 93, 94, 95, 96, 97, 98, 103, 104
  measures of, 22–24, 23t
  psychological or perceived, 8–9
  -resistance resources, 83
  see also stressors

stressors, 5, 8–11, 26, 27, 39, 42, 43, 58, 80, 81, 82, 83
subjective burden, 9, 17, 22, 23, 52–53

"tend-and-befriend" model, 58
transactional stress and coping model, 8–9, 42

unmitigated agency, 56–57, 59
unmitigated communion, 56–57, 59

Vilchinsky, N., 31, 86, 88

"we-disease", 29, 55
wear and tear hypothesis, 21–22
well-being of caregivers, 14, 16, 24, 34, 40, 46, 51–54, 67, 76, 83, 85, 91, 92, 95, 96, 101
  emotional, 9, 18, 26, 30, 32, 39, 53, 76
  mental, 31, 43, 100
  physical, 9, 76
  psychological, 19, 21, 60
  relational, 26, 29
  subjective, 51
Willingness to Care scale, 74
women caregivers, *see* female caregivers
  and burden, 52–53
  and childcare, 18, 55, 58
  and employment patterns, 54
  and identity, 57, 58, 59, 61
  and interpersonal relationships, 56–59
  and motivations for caregiving, 54–56
  relationship of caregiver to patient, 59–62
  social support and emotional disclosure, 58–59
  stress of, 50–52, 63
  unmitigated communion of, 57

Zarit Burden Interview, 22–23

The manufacturer's authorised representative in the EU is Springer Nature Customer Service Centre GmbH, Europaplatz 3, 69115 Heidelberg, Germany. If you have any concerns regarding our products, please contact ProductSafety@springernature.com

Printed and bound by CPI Group (UK) Ltd, Croydon, CR0 4YY

23/03/2026

02076402-0020